MOSES MAIMONIDES
ON THE CAUSES OF SYMPTOMS

MAQĀLAH FĪ BAYĀN BAʻḌ AL-AʻRĀḌ WA-AL-JAWĀB ʻANHĀ

MAʼAMAR HA-HAḴRAʻAH

DE CAUSIS ACCIDENTIUM

Edited by

J. O. LEIBOWITZ and S. MARCUS

In collaboration with

M. BEIT-ARIÉ, E. D. GOLDSCHMIDT,
F. KLEIN-FRANKE, E. LIEBER, M. PLESSNER

UNIVERSITY OF CALIFORNIA PRESS
BERKELEY   LOS ANGELES   LONDON

University of California Press
Berkeley and Los Angeles, California

University of California Press, Ltd.
London, England

Copyright © 1974, by
The Regents of the University of California

ISBN 0–520–02224–6

LC 71–187873

Printed in the United States of America

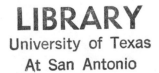

TABLE OF CONTENTS

Preface — J. O. Leibowitz   7

Introduction — J. O. Leibowitz   9

The Medical Contents of the Treatise — J. O. Leibowitz   19

A Palaeographic Description of the Jerusalem
Hebrew Manuscript — M. Beit-Arié   34

The Hebrew Text (Hebrew MS. Jerusalem 3941) with Corrections and Annotations
by S. Marcus   39
English Translation of the Treatise — A. Bar-Sela, H. E. Hoff and E. Faris   41
Running Commentary — J. O. Leibowitz   41

The Extant Arabic Manuscripts — M. Plessner   155

The Arabic Text (reproduced from Kroner's edition)   165

The Medieval Latin Translations:
Expanded Transcript of the Florence Incunable (The First Eighteen chapters of
the Treatise — E. D. Goldschmidt   189
The Hitherto Unpublished Part of the Latin Text (Chapter Nineteen to the End) —
F. Klein-Franke   198

Illustrations   after 200

The Materia Medica of the Treatise — S. Marcus   213

Bibliography   249

Index   259

PREFACE

EARLY in my career I became interested in the present treatise by Maimonides. At my suggestion, a beautiful reproduction of the Latin incunable of Maimonides' *Regimen* was published by my late friend Dr. Herbert Grossberger (Heidelberg, 1931). Most intriguing was the final section, later called "De causis accidentium," which the early Florentine printer had appended to the *Regimen* in a fragmentary way. Only a few pages of the medieval Hebrew translations of this section were known to scholars.

The situation changed when an almost complete thirteenth century manuscript of a Hebrew translation was discovered in 1962. A preliminary study of this text was carried out by Beverly A. Spirt (now Mrs. Marmor), under my supervision and with the help of Shlomo Marcus. This resulted in a thesis for the degree of Bachelor of Arts at Harvard (1967), which bears the title "A preliminary study of the Hebrew text of a Medical Treatise by Maimonides." It has been extensively used during the preparation of this volume, and I am indebted to Beverly Marmor for this contribution.

The next acknowledgments are to my regular collaborators. I am much indebted to Shlomo Marcus, who has given much of his time and of his vast knowledge to the achievement of our goal. Besides providing a full catalogue of materia medica, he acted as coordinator of our team and identified himself with each phase and facet of the project. A learned librarian and multilingual, he has succeeded in unearthing valuable information from little-known sources, including manuscripts. For the past few years we have had the privilege of having Elinor Lieber on our staff. I am much indebted to her for tracing sources, chiefly in Galenic writings, in order to explain certain passages in our treatise. She helped us in elucidating the medical implications of the texts, in the production and editing of the essays, commentaries and translations, and graciously watched over the English style throughout the volume.

Among the guest contributors to this edition I would like to express my thanks to Professor Martin Plessner for his advice on Arabic and general matters. Professor Plessner's participation in our weekly staff conferences over the years was always very stimulating, and I appreciated his readiness to answer our questions. He kindly helped us to avoid pitfalls, when some of our tentative conjectures did not withstand the criterion of sound philological insight. A renowned scholar in his field, he has provided an essay on the Arabic manuscripts of our treatise. During some of our conferences we also had the benefit of advice from David Tené, an expert in medieval Hebrew. Early in our work, Malachi Beit-Arié was our adviser on the palaeographic aspects of the Hebrew manuscript. I thank him for this and for his concise and revealing essay. Felix Klein-Franke undertook the pioneering task of preparing a critical edition of that part of the Latin manuscripts which is lacking in the incunable and the sixteenth century printed versions; we much appreciate his work on this as well as his introductory essay. The writer is a Latinist as well as an Arabic scholar; a combination of qualities befitting the synthetic character of this volume. The late Dr. Ernst Daniel Goldschmidt was kind enough to expand the abbreviations in the incunable of the Latin translation of the treatise.

I would also like to acknowledge the valuable help of the following persons and institutions: The National and University Library, Jerusalem for permission to reproduce the Hebrew text, and its staff members for their assistance; the American Philosophical Society for permission to reproduce the English translation of the treatise; Dr. Ariel Bar-Sela for his kind advice and for the photostat of the manuscript of an early Latin translation; Ilay Ilan for his advice on Arabic philology; Professor Moshe Prywes, chief editor of the *Israel Journal of Medical Sciences*, for his inspiration; Mrs. Shula Toledano, manager of the *Journal*, for her gracious help in making the publication of this volume possible; Mr. Ernst Jacob for seeing the book through the press; and Dr. David V. Zaitchek for his advice on plant identification.

The list of thanks would be incomplete should we forget Harry Friedenwald of Baltimore, who died in 1950. By the bequest of his collection to the Hebrew University Library, Dr. Friedenwald laid the foundations of medico-historical activity at this university. Indeed, most of our work was carried out in the Friedenwald Collection room.

Last but not least, I wish to express my thanks to the National Library of Medicine for the grant which has made possible the appearance of this volume. The policy followed by this library calls to mind the somewhat similar activity of the Royal Society of London in the seventeenth and eighteenth centuries, when the Society demonstrated its humanitarian and universal outlook by generously sponsoring the publication of scholarly editions of works of foreign authors.

J. O. Leibowitz

Hebrew University–Hadassah Medical School
Jerusalem, Israel

Prof. M. Plessner died on November 27. 1973. after this volume was completed in press.

INTRODUCTION

J. O. LEIBOWITZ

THE INCENTIVE for the present work was the chance discovery in the early 1960s of a hitherto unknown Hebrew translation of this treatise of Maimonides, when a collection of 115 Hebrew manuscripts was acquired from the estate of R. Hayyim Bekor ha-Levi by the Jewish National and University Library of Jerusalem. Among these was a bound volume of four medical works by Maimonides, Jerusalem 8° 3941, including the late thirteenth-century manuscript which is reproduced and edited in this volume (see Beit-Arié, 1962–1963).

In general, the early Hebrew and Latin translations of the medical works of Maimonides greatly help toward the understanding of the original Arabic texts. However, previous editors and translators of this treatise have only been able to compare the Arabic text with fragments of the Hebrew manuscripts of the work (Berlin 232, fols. 116v to 119r, now kept in Tübingen, and Munich 280, fol. 134). Our present manuscript is far more extensive, although it lacks a short passage in the middle and a second following page 154v, and the entire last chapter is missing, so that it ends abruptly.

Stimulated by the discovery of this Hebrew version, we realized that a more detailed study of the contents would be rewarding. This was achieved with the cooperation of experts in the fields of Arabic, Hebrew, and Latin philology. Their assistance was required not only on account of the linguistic problems involved, but also for the reproduction of our Hebrew text and of a Latin version of the last part of the work, which comprises more than half of the entire treatise. This part of the Latin text, from Chapter 19 onward, is reproduced here, because it is missing in the printed Latin editions of the author's *Regimen of Health*, to all of which our treatise was appended (Florence, c. 1477; Pavia, 1501; Venice, 1514 and 1521; Augsburg, 1518; and Lyons, 1535).

Although *De causis accidentium* is associated with the *Regimen* in the Latin editions, there is no doubt that these were entirely separate treatises. In his introduction to the *Regimen*, Maimonides states that this work will be divided into four chapters. The fourth chapter ends with a phrase indicating that the work is now concluded: "This is the measure of what the servant has now presented for the needs of our Master, may God perpetuate his dominion for him unto all times." Moreover, in the introductory phrase of *De causis accidentium*, Maimonides gives his reasons for addressing a second treatise to the same Sultan al-Afdal. However, because of the identity of the addressee and the relative brevity of the second work, the two treatises were usually printed together.

The omission in the printed versions of some seven-tenths of the text can possibly be attributed to the example of the first printed edition, that of Florence, c. 1477, "apud sanctum Iacobum de Ripolis." The story of the printing press at this convent may cast some light on the subject (see Haebler, 1924, p. 157). Its beginnings were very modest. The work was carried out by nuns under the supervision of senior monks, who called on Johannes Petri, a German professional printer, to run the press. It is to be noted that the unprinted part of the manuscript starts with a comment by Maimonides that he "has now responded to all sections of that noble letter" and contains the remark that the contents about to follow have already "been mentioned in preceding paragraphs." It is thus likely that those at the press were glad to be able to economize and dispense with printing the rest of the manuscript. This first edition seems to have set the pattern for its successors, insofar as the text was amputated at the same spot each time.

The next edition of the work, printed in Pavia in 1501, *in folio*, is incorporated together with the *Regimen* in the *Tabula consiliorum* of J. M. Ferrarius de Gradibus. Here our treatise has been given (fol. "p.d.") the typographical form of a new chapter, but has not been expressly numbered as such. It has also received a title of its own: *De causis accidentium*[1] *apparentium domino et magnifico soldano et de temporibus apparitionis eorum* (On the causes of happenings [medically: symptoms] which have become manifest to the Master and magnificent Sultan and of the time of their appearance). The excipit is as in the first edition: Laus deo et Marie virgini.

The third edition, Venice, 1514, is again included in the collection of consilia issued by Ferrarius de Gradibus. It presents a new feature, the combined work being entitled *Tractatus quinque*, and so on (fol. 105a). Our treatise now constitutes the fifth tractate, and its title remains as given in the Pavia version (fol. 109b). The text ends with the same religious formula as the previous edition.

Both treatises were printed in Augsburg in 1518, in the form of five "tractates." This time however, they appeared as an independent small volume, our treatise starting on page "d." No religious formula was appended. The last Latin printing was in Lyons, in 1535, again in a collection of consilia. Our treatise bears the same caption as the Venice edition and ends with the same benediction, first found in the Florence incunable.

In retrospect, the early sixteenth-century editions closely follow the text of the incunable, although captions have been added, abbreviations somewhat expanded, and very slight changes introduced in the wording. These editions appear to have

---

[1] In both Arabic and Hebrew, the word corresponding to "accidens" denotes a happening, or a case of disease. In late Latin, the word may also denote: "Morbus, infortunium." See Du Cange, 1883 edition, I: 46, *s.v.* 2. Accidentia.

been modeled on the text of the incunable rather than on that of a manuscript. A further hint to this effect is the invocation of the Virgin Mary in the final benediction; in the Venice 1514 edition of the very long work by Ferrarius de Gradibus which immediately precedes the Maimonides treatise, the formula is "Laus dei semper."

Of the four extant Latin manuscripts, three were consulted by us: Vatican MS. Palatine Latin 1298; Vienna MS. Cod. Latin 5306; and Friedenwald 572. The last is included in a volume of Latin translations of six medical treatises of Maimonides in the Friedenwald Collection in Jerusalem (see Friedenwald, 1946, p. 99). Manuscript Vienna Cod. Latin 2280 was not examined, because we have not aimed at presenting all variants of the Latin text. We have however, included the text of the incunable (with the original abbreviations expanded) and have supplemented this incomplete text with the missing portion, taken from the manuscripts.

Steinschneider (1893, pp. 772–774) was the first to make an examination of our treatise. He suggested that it may have been translated into Latin by John of Capua, the converted Jew who translated the *Regimen* at some time during the thirteenth century. Steinschneider believed that John of Capua translated exclusively from the Hebrew and therefore felt that a Hebrew version of the combined work must once have been in existence (Steinschneider, 1893, p. 773). If the translation were indeed made from the Hebrew, this would somewhat diminish its authenticity, but its early date in any case ensures its reliability with regard to notions and definitions current at that time.

The Hebrew versions have been briefly mentioned in the opening paragraphs of this introduction. We have already noted that the newly-discovered Jerusalem manuscript was not known to previous scholars. Even as early as the thirteenth century, the work must have been so rare that the scribe felt impelled to add a marginal note at the beginning of his transcript: "This [treatise] is missing from the books of the physician." One can sense the relief of the scribe in having finally found the treatise to which other scribes appeared to have alluded in various versions of the *Regimen*. For example, in MS. Berlin 72 of the *Regimen*, the copyist adds: "This is to be followed by the 'Book of Decision' [*Ma'amar ha-Hakra'ah:* the title given by the scribe to our treatise] which I have in another volume", and so on. The search for this rare work is given more poignant expression by the fifteenth-century Hebrew scribe, who had at his disposal only a few fragments of the manuscript (MS. Berlin 232, see above) and added: "Behold, this is all that I have found from the great rabbi, Rabbi Moses of blessed memory. My soul sought more but I did not find it." Here a longer caption for the work *De causis accidentium* has been provided by the scribe: "Responses of Maimonides of great purport to special questions posed by a certain king; in order that he should decide (*le-hakri'a*) between conflicting opinions of the doctors. Some of these have been written down here with God's help."

Since Maimonides himself gave no caption to our treatise, and each of the various scribes provided his own, the Latin title, *De causis accidentium*, first given to the early sixteenth-century editions, became generally adopted. It is derived from the wording of the fourth line of the first paragraph of the incunable, folio **ei**, which corresponds to the unnumbered page 65 of the complete volume, on which our treatise starts.

The headings given to the works of Maimonides, both medical and others, often originate from the wording of the opening paragraphs, prefaces, or epistles which preceded the main texts. Thus the name of his religious code, *Mishneh Torah* (which incidentally was not accepted in daily use), is given at the end of a long preface, immediately preceding the first of the fourteen books of the work. In the case of his philosophical work known as *The Guide for the Perplexed*, the title is located in a letter of Maimonides written in Hebrew to his pupil Joseph ben Judah. No mention of it is found in the somewhat similar dedicatory letter in Arabic, although the word "perplexed" appears (Baneth, 1946, pp. 6–16).

The heading of Maimonides' chief medical work, *The Aphorisms*, is probably based on the first lines of the preface, in which the author notes that the literary form was taken from the *Aphorisms* of Hippocrates and the contents were "chosen from all the works of Galen." It was thus a simple matter for later scribes to name the work "The Aphorisms of Moses" (*Aphorismi Moyses*, Bologna, 1489). Lastly, in the *Regimen sanitatis*, to which our *De causis accidentium* was usually appended, the word "regimen" is already used in the opening lines, and the first chapter is headed "On the Regimen of Health in General." In this way the titles may have come into existence, irrespective of whether they were used by Maimonides himself. As far as the Hebrew versions are concerned, there is no doubt that the titles were added by the translators or scribes.

The original Arabic text came to the attention of scholars much later than the Latin versions. It was first published by Hermann Kroner (1870–1930), in *Janus*, 1928, where it was accompanied by a preface, a translation into German, the text of the Hebrew fragments, and a critical apparatus. This edition will be discussed below by Martin Plessner, in his review of the Arabic sources. Kroner's pioneering effort to present scholarly editions of some of the medical works of Maimonides was achieved despite his relative isolation as rabbi of Bopfingen, a small German country town (see Marcus, 1971). It brings to mind the work of Francis Adams (1796–1861), who translated and edited Greek medical texts while carrying on his work as a busy practitioner in an isolated Scottish area.

A more recent German edition with a preface and notes was issued by Suessmann Muntner in 1966. In 1969 the same author published his own translation of the work into Hebrew, under the title *Medical Responses*.

The Arabic specialists on our team have consulted the relevant manuscripts in this language, including MS. Paris 1211, written in Arabic in Hebrew characters. This source was only used in part by previous editors and translators. We are grateful to Ernest Mainz who, together with the staff of the Bibliothèque Nationale, Paris, succeeded in putting into order misplaced leaves in the bound copy.

The treatise and the *Regimen* have been translated together from the Arabic into English by Bar-Sela, Hoff, and Faris and published in the *Transactions of the American Philosophical Society* for 1964. Their translation is incorporated in this volume. A certain number of divergent readings and interpretations, some of them based on the authority of MS. Paris 1211, have been noted with the consent of the above-named translators. It is to be understood that although the English translation appears in this volume facing the Hebrew text, it refers solely to the Arabic original, which is also reproduced here.

In view of the availability of this translation from the Arabic, we did not consider it justifiable to provide an English version of the Jerusalem Hebrew text. The language of this Hebrew version is quite unusual, differing not only from that used in Hebrew poetry but also from that of other medieval medical translators, such as the Tibbonids or Nathan ha-Me'ati. It is particularly close to the Arabic and contains a number of new Hebrew words formed along Arabic patterns.

In the course of producing this critical edition of a Maimonides text, we have kept in mind the wider issues, especially the question of transmission of the Greek medical heritage. Thus our study would fit into the framework of present-day research on the transmission of ancient science and medicine through the Middle Ages. In some instances we have compared the ideas of Maimonides with those of Hippocrates and Galen. We have also tried, as far as possible, to locate the references to these authors which are specifically mentioned in the treatise. The task is made more difficult by the fact that we do not know which of the Arabic translations of the works of Galen and Hippocrates were used by Maimonides. In those cases in which the name of the work is given by Maimonides but the quotation cannot be identified, we are led to suspect that he used a version different from our present standard texts.

The share of Maimonides in the transmission of Greek medicine was the extraction of relevant doctrines and facts from the great mass of Hippocratic and Galenic writings. Not pretending to be original, Maimonides manifested his own view and approach by his discriminating choice of the material handed down from antiquity, as he himself points out in the preface to his *Aphorisms*. Our small treatise demonstrates his ability to apply this knowledge to his own practice, as well as to commit it to paper in a concise and readable manner. From ancient sources[2] he acquired his special interest in the "constitution" of the individual patient. On the other hand, in a treatise of this intent and scope, we cannot expect to find any criticism leading to a rejection of older theories. Such criticism does occur in his more general works, such as the *Aphorisms*, where he occasionally rejects Galen's views, or in

---

[2] Cf. Hippocrates, *On ancient medicine*, end of Chapter 20; in the Jones edition, I: 55.

his *Commentary on the Aphorisms of Hippocrates*, in which he denies the validity of some of the latter's aphorisms.

Although rooted in the Galenic tradition, some medical and physiological ideas of Maimonides reveal original facets, insofar as he stresses particular points which are only vaguely referred to by Galen and formulates others in his own way. This applies for example, to various scattered observations about the blood which are found in our treatise and which call for analysis and interpretation. Thus, Maimonides mentions "that a vessel had once been opened and there came out blood as thick as spleen, whereupon the physicians counseled on this account, further bloodletting" (142r, 10–13).[3] Significantly, he comments: "What should be aimed at always is clarification of the blood"; probably he meant by this that the blood should be made thinner. We would not go so far as to suppose that Maimonides was fully aware of the concept of polycythemia, a condition discovered very much later, but his introduction of this topic is quite remarkable. We have searched for Galenic parallels but failed to find any convincing description of this condition. Galen's indications for bloodletting are mainly for "abundance" of the blood, as for example, in *De sanitate tuenda*, Book VI, Chapter 13, (K. VI: 443). However, no phrase "blood as thick as spleen" is used there. Moreover, our impression on reading these passages is that Galen was referring to a hemodynamic rather than a hematological disorder.[4]

Other passages in Galen on "thickness of the blood" seem even to connote thrombotic phenomena. Such an impression is obtained on reading his *De differentiis febrium*, Book II, Chapter 11 (K. VII: 375), where he points to "corruption of the blood clotted in the small vessels," a Galenic idea of great moment. Elsewhere we have drawn attention to Galen's actual use of the word "thrombosis" (Leibowitz, 1970, p. 126). However, this fine Galenic observation is not identical with that in our treatise.

One of the Galenic ideas on the blood which Maimonides has taken over unchanged is that blood is produced by the liver. Accordingly he advises "clarification of the blood and rectification of the temperament of the liver, so that good blood be generated" (142v, 3–4), for which purpose he had already recommended special syrups in the *Regimen*. An expression such as "praiseworthy blood, of the nature of the natural blood" (134r, 9–10) is similar to Galen's "sanguis bonus" (*Hipp. de acut. morb. victu comm.* IV; K. XV: 883), or "optimus" (*De atra bile*, Chapter 2; K. V: 107).

An important concept discussed by Maimonides is that of water-balance and hemoconcentration in hot countries. He first describes sweat as a manifestation of "vapors that ascend to the surface of the body" (141r, 1–2). From here he proceeds

---

3 Here and subsequently the references are to the pages and lines of the Hebrew text. See introduction, p. 17.

4 In Book IV, Chapter 15 of *De usu partium* (K. III: 319–320), Galen states: "The blood attracted to the spleen is thicker than that in the liver . . . the liver is nourished by useful, thick blood" (see May translation, 1968, I: 234).

to consider the effect of hot regions on a pathological condition, in which the vapors "arise from thick turbid blood . . . and . . . augment the thickness of the blood" (141r, 3–4). Maimonides therefore forbids his patient to travel to hot regions, to prevent worsening of his possibly polycythemic condition. The influence of external heat on the functions of the body is already mentioned by Hippocrates (*The Sacred Disease*, Chapter 13), but without reference to the composition of the blood. A passage in Galen's *De consuetudinis* (Daremberg, I: 105) is devoted to the influence of heat on the body and mentions "dry and wet heat," but the passage lacks the physiological insight into water-balance which is implied by Maimonides.

The word "vapors" also occurs in other parts of the treatise. On page 136r, 6, we find a reference to "generation of black vapors caused by the black bile arising from the combustion of phlegm that recurs periodically." Here, the "vapors" seem to represent some metabolic end-products. Earlier, on page 133v, 4, they figure in the phrase: ". . . aid the egress of the superfluities by promoting a copious flow of urine and expel from the blood the smoky vapors." Thus some of the "superfluities" or noxious agents are eliminated through the urine (133v, 5–6) — a kind of clearance as understood and measured in modern medical tests. The use of the words "superfluities" or "smoky vapors" would fit into the Galenic ideas of "residues" (see p. 20).

As in his better-known works, Maimonides is very attentive to the psychology of his patient. All his lesser suggestions, such as agreeable company, music, and so on, which are found in our treatise, conform with this outspoken dictum, given in the third chapter of his *Regimen:* "concern and care shall always be given to the movements of the psyche; these should be kept in balance in the state of health as well as in disease, and no other regimen should be given precedence in any wise." In the same chapter, the influence of the "movements of the soul" on the body have been forcefully delineated. In expressions similar to those adopted by Maimonides, Galen mentions death induced by anger or by excessive pleasure (*De locis affectis*, Book V. Chapter 2; K. VIII: 301–302; Daremberg, II: 627). This is but one of the passages which show that Galen was clearly aware of the influence of the soul on the body. However, Maimonides elevates the subject of emotion and disease to a leading principle of therapeutics and integrates it into his system of medicine.

Conscious of the great influence of the mind on the state of the body, Maimonides suggested in the *Regimen* some kind of psychotherapy to quiet the emotions. In our treatise he also proposes the use of certain drugs which he believes to be effective for this purpose. The first indication is the melancholy disposition of the Sultan, for which he advises an extract of the plant popularly known as oxtongue. "If the oxtongue is steeped in wine, it increases the dilation and the delight of the spirit" (133v, 14–16). Oxtongue taken in wine is recommended by a number of ancient authors, among them Dioscorides (IV, 126 [128]). Secondly, Maimonides expands this indication to certain cardiac conditions, which we now associate with particular

15

manifestations of coronary disease, collapse, and its mitigated form "lipothymia."
Here the oxtongue is added to a great number of other ingredients (148r, 13–14).
Maimonides seems to have a high opinion of its potency: "When the physicians
speak of the drink that exhilarates, in general they mean the syrup of oxtongue"
(133v, 11–14). Little was known until recently about the pharmacological action of
this plant (*Anchusa officinalis*), which Maimonides thought to exert a psychotropic
action (see the running commentary to 133r, line 8 on page 51).

An unusual feature of this treatise, which is not found in other medical works of
Maimonides, is the inclusion of a long quotation from another author, beginning
on page 145r, 9, of the Hebrew manuscript. This is a very detailed prescription
from *De viribus cordis* by Ibn Sina, a work which is appended to several Latin
editions of the *Canon* and which exists also in Hebrew translations, of which we used
MSS. Munich 280 and 87. Two medical indications are given for the so-called
"jacinth electuary" (145r, 9–10): cardiac manifestations (for example, 145v, 1), and
"melancholia, a disorder that tends towards mania" (147r, 4). The different conditions are treated by "adding to and taking from it [the basic formula] according
to each and every temperament" (145r, 16–17). Thus a special formula is provided
for those who "are attacked by palpitation and weakness of the heart because of
the badness of their hot temperament" (147r, 10–11). The linkage of mind and body
in this prescription of Ibn Sina would have been in tune with the medical outlook
of Maimonides. It is possible that this was the reason why he quoted the passage
verbatim.

It may be felt that the inclusion of this long prescription somewhat disturbs the
literary balance of the composition. In fact, Maimonides did not intend this work
to be a formal treatise. Its scope and form were governed by the practical considerations involved in acting as an arbiter between the divergent opinions of the other
court physicians. It comes under the classification of the so-called "consilia," which
concerned a particular subject or patient and were popular in the West in the late
Middle Ages and the Renaissance. We have already noted that it was included as
such in a Latin collection of consilia, printed several times between 1480 and 1535.
More about consilia is to be found in P. Laín Entralgo's informative book, *La
historia clinica* (1950). This literary form is reflected in the Hebrew title (*The Book
of Decision*) given to the treatise by the translator (see above).

In his replies, Maimonides is on the whole outspoken and does not hesitate to
refute the opinions of his colleagues when necessary. In most cases he acknowledges
the rationale of their advice but finds that it does not correspond with the case or
the constitution of the patient. On one occasion he takes the opportunity to censure
those physicians who neglect the study of the digestive organs (138r, 2–6), although
"the best physicians have devoted treatises to it." He then presents his general views
on the working of the stomach in health and in disease and considers the effects of
diet and medication on its tonus and secretion and on the degree of "viscidity of

the phlegm." He admonishes the doctors for failing to consider "whether the stomach is debilitated or not and whether there is moistness in it or not" (138*r*, 13 to 138*v*, 2). Maimonides thus demonstrates a pathophysiological approach to the problem, without trying to isolate individual diseases not sufficiently known in his time.

Although the treatise is only designed to provide an answer to specific questions regarding an individual patient, Maimonides in fact succeeds in discussing a number of different medical subjects. Scattered throughout the treatise are some of his views on problems of the circulatory system, the digestive organs and general dietetics, psychiatry, and specific aspects of physiology. All these matters are discussed in the essay which follows this introduction and which deals with the medical contents of the treatise. The points are considered according to the order of their appearance in the twenty-two chapters of the text.

A special feature of this volume is a running commentary which accompanies the text of the treatise. This is based on the Hebrew version, which has here been edited and published for the first time. However, in any case of divergence from the Arabic original, the latter has been given full preference. In some respects we have tried to emulate Francis Adams, who appended a detailed commentary to his translations of the *Aphorisms* of Hippocrates and of the works of Paulus Aegineta.

The purpose of our commentary is to facilitate understanding of the medical meaning of the treatise. In addition to the critical philological evaluation, we therefore introduce a somewhat new approach to the presentation of an old medical text, trying, wherever possible, to explain the words and notions hidden behind an obscure terminology. In some instances we have been able to interpret enigmatic portions of the text in the light of modern knowledge. Finally, we have succeeded in tracing the origin of certain assertions and ideas of Maimonides to more ancient sources.

This introduction is followed by an essay on the medical contents of the work and then by a palaeographic evaluation of the Hebrew manuscript. These introduce the Hebrew and English texts, which are printed facing one another. The lower part of these pages is occupied by a running commentary and corrections to the Hebrew text. Preceding the Arabic text is an essay on the extant Arabic manuscripts. The next part of the work concerns the Latin translations. It consists first of an expanded transcript of the incunable. This is followed by an introductory essay to the next section: an edition of the portion of the Latin text which is missing in the incunable, accompanied by a critical apparatus. The volume ends with a catalogue of the materia medica of the treatise. The pagination of the texts in all four languages (130*v* to 156*v*) corresponds to that of the Hebrew manuscript.

For the first time the manifold facets of a Maimonides text are brought together in one multilingual edition. This fact, as well as the inclusion of specialized essays will, we hope, make this volume acceptable to a wider range of readers than would be a medical text of the past issued in the customary form.

THE MEDICAL CONTENTS OF THE TREATISE

J. O. LEIBOWITZ

THE TREATISE takes the form of the consilia of the Middle Ages and Renaissance (see Sudhoff, 1922, pp. 202–204): that is, a detailed response to specific questions arising out of medical practice. Such a format is not suitable for a lengthy presentation of general ideas and principles. It does however, provide an opportunity for the author to display his individual approach toward the patient in question and his medical attitude to the problems directly involved in the particular case, without too much generalization or the elaboration of medical theories.

An example of this is found in the first chapter of the treatise, in the discussion on the need for medical intervention in the case of an attack of piles. In general, according to Maimonides, this should be left to nature, because "when Nature opens these vessels, she opens them in the required measure" (131v, 10–13). However, intervention is justified if "those places are swollen, and the pain is greatly increased" (132v, 11). But the author adds: "Then we open them by medication so that whatever was dispelled there from the blood and caused those places to swell flows out" (132v, 11–14). Here the author has attempted to explain the underlying cause, in this case, the blood which had congested in the anal veins.

The next discussion is in Chapter 2 and concerns the "dilation of the spirit" produced by the administration of a vinous extract of the herb oxtongue, apparently for its psychotropic effects. This preparation is mentioned by Dioscorides (Book IV, 126 [128]), as well as by other authors, including Galen and Avicenna. The indications are discussed at length. In addition to piles and constipation, the king seems to have suffered from a depressive mental state, a condition which Maimonides, like earlier authors, attributes to the effect of black bile. The extract of oxtongue in wine is also called here "the drink that exhilarates" (133v, 12). According to the author it exerts general effects; it "moistens the body" (134r) and "generates praiseworthy blood, of the nature of the natural blood, which is hot and wet" (134r, 9–11).

The stress laid by Maimonides on the use of this preparation demonstrates his earnest attempt to treat mental symptoms. But it was not easy to explain the pharmacological action of the preparation until new light was shed on the problem by chemical and animal investigations carried out in 1970 (see the running commentary, 133r on p. 51). The idea that the plant "generates praiseworthy blood" was probably common in the Middle Ages (Avicenna, Ibn al-Bayṭār).

The ancient and medieval physicians were not greatly concerned with hematology, so that even a side remark of this kind is worthy of note. However, in this section Maimonides is primarily interested in the action of the drug in "effacing the black humor and eradicating its traces" (134*v*, 13–14). Of greater hematological significance are his remarks concerning "thick turbid blood" in his discussion of the effects on the body of a hot climate (Chapter 12, pp. 22–23).

With regard to "the drink that exhilarates," Maimonides distinguishes between its intrinsic effects and those of the wine with which it may be mixed. He further notes the properties of the tincture that are produced by steeping pieces of the bark in wine for twelve hours.

The administration of oxtongue in a mixture with other medicaments is also mentioned in Chapter III of the *Regimen of Health* (Muntner Hebrew edition, pp. 54 f.; Bar-Sela English translation, pp. 23–24) where it is said, among other actions, to "dilate the soul" and to "strengthen the heart." Such an association of psychic and cardiac effects has already been briefly discussed in the introduction (p. 16). It is interesting that the thirteenth century herbalist Rufinus also recommends a particular drug as a remedy "contra cardiacam et sincopim" as well as "contra melancholicam passionem" (see Leibowitz, 1970, p. 44). With regard to the properties of the wine alone, these are detailed in the *Regimen* (Chapter IV), where its negative aspect— the production of a state of drunkenness—is mentioned and it is noted that wine is harmful for the young but good for the old.

In Chapter 3 of our treatise (135*r*, 13 ff.), the case of the Sultan is reviewed in the light of the humoral theory. His temperament was considered to tend "toward the hot one," with "the generation of black vapors caused by the black bile arising from the combustion of phlegm that recurs periodically" (136*r*, 5–6). The author therefore rejects the medicaments recommended by the other doctors, which he claims are suitable only "for one who is dominated by yellow bile" (Hebrew: "red bile"; 136*r*, 1).

Unlike the other three humors, black bile does not appear to represent a physiological fluid, but is rather a hypothetical product of the body metabolism. For example, Galen states: "The spleen is the organ which repels the black bile (atrabilis) which is produced in the liver" (*De usu partium*, Book IV, 15; K. III: 321). In Chapter 2 of the treatise, Maimonides speaks of harmful substances which are removed from the body by the urine in the course of metabolism which "expel from the blood the smoky vapors" (133*v*, 4–7). The expression "smoky vapors" is similar to the term "lignyōdes peritōma" ("excrementa fuliginosa") used by Galen in the above passage, as well as to the "fumosa fuliginosa" of *De methodo medendi*, Book VIII, Chapter 4 (K. X: 566).

Chapter 4 deals with the use of rhubarb (rhabarber, *Rheum*) in the treatment of constipation. Maimonides suggests drinking it "one day and then abstaining for two," presumably in order to prevent habit formation. The subject of purgatives is dealt with separately and in more detail in Chapter 13, beginning at 141r, 9.

Chapter 5 on bathing, exercising, and anointing the body with oil is also very short, four lines in all. This is a further sign that the treatise was only intended to indicate opinions diverging from those of the other doctors consulted. Otherwise the author relies on the views expressed in his *Regimen of Health*—which was addressed to the same Sultan—and he does not feel that it is necessary to repeat or expand them.

In Chapter 6 the author rejects any medicament which is not consonant with the particular condition of the patient. Thus, the Sultan is clearly not in need of treatment for "the intensely inflaming burning fevers." Again, Maimonides opposes the suggestion that the Sultan be required to drink fresh milk (Hebrew: "milk fresh from the cow"; 137r, 4), because he believes that the main cause of the symptoms is "inflamed phlegm" (white bile) and that such milk has the property of "quick transformation into any humor whatever" (137r, 5–6).

Chapter 7 (137r, 9 ff.) deals with the effects of some particular drugs on the digestive processes in the stomach. The author notes that there is a difference between taking a drug on an empty stomach and taking it after a meal; but he is against prescribing barberry extract at any time, possibly because it increases the gastric acidity.

In Chapter 8 the author returns to the subject of "the exhilarating drink" to which are added various medicaments, such as *rumex* (sorrel) and *melissa*, the psychopharmacological effects of which if any, are not known. He does, however, note that fleabane (*Plantago psyllium L.*) should not be prescribed, presumably because it is toxic if taken in excess. (See the running commentary for 137v, 13). *Melissa officinalis L.* (balm gentle) is discussed at length by Ibn al-Bayṭār (Sontheimer, I: 108–109), who particularly quotes Avicenna to the effect that "it rejoices the heart and reduces the black bile."

In Chapter 9 the author stresses the importance of the functions of the stomach and advises physicians not to neglect its study but to pay special attention to this organ, "as the best physicians are said to have done" (138r, 5). This is one of the rare pleas for the study of gastroenterology to be found in early medicohistorical literature. The chapter consists largely of a polemic against adding "poppy and seeds of round pumpkin" to barley water. Maimonides favors the use of barley water as a gastric remedy, in the tradition of Hippocrates, who prescribed it repeatedly (see below, p. 32). He considers the effects of the recommended mixture on two main aspects of gastric function: tonus and mucus secretion ("catarrh") (138v, 1 and 7–11). This can be inferred from his statement that the mixture will indeed "strengthen the stomach . . . [and] dry its moisture." He claims, however, that these beneficial properties may be nullified when harmful substances such as opium are added to the mixture. He is opposed to the polypragmasia of the other doctors, who induce constipation with opium and then give prunes to correct it.

21

Chapter 10 deals with the last course of the main meal. It should be noted that it is customary in the Near East to remain at table for some time after the main part of the meal is over; nonalcoholic beverages are then drunk and large quantities of various seeds and fruits are eaten. Maimonides objects to the eating of coriander seeds which, although still used as a condiment, may give rise to nausea and even vomiting when taken alone. He maintains that they should be prescribed as a medicament in powder form and preferably cooked with the food. He does however, recommend the consumption of purslane seeds in sugar because of their power of "cooling and strengthening the heart."

Chapter 11 is devoted to the fruit to be eaten after the meal. The author is generally opposed to "fresh fruits" being "taken as nutrients," presumably meaning in large quantities. Only "if there was need to induce appetite, or a habit of taking fruits," does he agree that "one should take before the meal whatever softens the stools and after the meal those fruits in which there is astringence" (140r, 4–6). He advises the Sultan "to avoid fresh fruits all he can" (140v, 5–6) and explains his veto of soft fruits, such as watermelon and apricots, "because of the rapidity of their change into whatever evil humor there is in the body" (140r, 13–14). Moreover, in the case of soft fruit, such as the peach, the "substance" of the fruit may give rise to "evil malignant fevers." However, the author believes that certain fruits are healthy, such as the "pear, quince, and apple" (140r, 7). These arguments are further developed at the end of Chapter I of the *Regimen of Health* and both here and in the *Regimen* Maimonides quotes Galen as saying that "since he stopped eating all fresh fruits, he had not had a fever to the end of his life" (see *De probis pravisque alimentorum succis*, Chapter I; K. VI: 755 ff.). Ibn Zuhr makes a similar statement in his "De nutrimentis,"[1] where he recommends only dates and grapes. Avicenna states that fruit is harmful if it is too juicy (Gruner edition, 1930, p. 375, § 759). The matter is clearly explained by Galen (*De alimentorum facultatibus*, Book II, Chapter 2; K. VI: 558 ff.), who states that "summer" fruits (which are mainly "soft" fruits) are particularly prone to go bad in hot weather and give rise to food poisoning. The likelihood of such infection was of course, increased by the poor sanitary conditions and the shortage of water in which to wash the fruit, especially those, such as watermelons, which grow close to the ground.

In Chapter 12, the author disapproves of eating game or "cured" meat since, according to the humoral theory, these exert a "heating" effect. The latter part of this chapter deals with the effects on the body of a hot climate, and the author appears to have some idea of the occurrence of hemoconcentration. He notes that excessive sweating may "augment the thickness of the blood," especially if the

---

[1] MS. Munich 220[1]. Hebrew translation probably by Nathan ha-Me'ati; see Steinschneider, 1893, p. 749.

patient already has "thick turbid blood" (141r, 3–4). Observations of this kind about the blood are rarely found in the medical literature of the Middle Ages.

In Chapter 13, Maimonides deals with various emetics and purgatives and is opposed to the use of strong medicaments of this kind. He draws attention to the fact that the excessive use of water lily "thickens the blood" (141v, 10), possibly through loss of fluid. Indeed, the fact that blood could be thicker than normal was known long before the nineteenth century, when the first methods were devised for counting the red blood cells. The author then notes that the action of a drug may be altered by the mode of administration. Thus dodder of thyme (*Cuscuta epithymum*) is harmful when cooked, but "if . . . infused in whey . . . it is good" (142r, 1–12). It should be given sparingly, at fifteen-day intervals, presumably to prevent any cumulative action. It is possible that any toxic effect of the alkaloids of this plant may be suppressed by a mixture with proteins of whey.

In Chapter 14, Maimonides displays a conservative attitude to venesection, as in his Code (*Mishneh Torah*). He limits his discussion on the subject to the particular condition of the Sultan, for which he considers that venesection is required, because "out came blood as thick as spleen" (142r, 11–12). This must have been a case of polycythemia, for which venesection is still performed today, to supplement the more modern form of treatment with radioactive phosphorus. He notes that venesection is indicated when a state of "plethora" occurs[2] (142r, 14). In the Hebrew translation, a more picturesque phrase is used, denoting "straining the blood" (142v, 3), as in the case of a turbid liquid which is filtered in order to cleanse and thin it. Galen speaks similarly of a deposit of black bile in the blood (*De temperamentis*, Book II, Chapter 3; K. I: 603).

The ancients believed that the blood was formed in the liver. This accounts for the phrase "rectification of the temperament of the liver so that good blood is generated" (142v, 3–4). (See also Galen, *De usu partium*, IV, 3; K. III: 269 f.). Maimonides notes (142v, 3–4) that "clarification of the blood" can be achieved not only be venesection but also by certain medicinal syrups, about which he has already spoken in the *Regimen of Health*, Chapter II, similarly in connection with venesection.

Chapter 15 contains instructions with regard to the diet in the summer, when one must be particularly careful "not to harm the stomach" (142v, 9) and thereby the balance of the humors. Thus in summer goat's meat should be prepared in such a manner that it will result in "the equilibration of the temperament" (143r, 2). For the same reason, "cooling concoctions" should not be freely prescribed even in summer (142v, 13 to 143r, 1).

In the author's opinion, "inflammation of the phlegm" (143r, 4) is the main cause

---

2 Cf. Galen *In Hippocratis Epidem. VI et Galeni in illum commentarius V*, Sectio V, Chapter 29 (K. XVIIB: 297): ". . . quibus sanguis crassus est, iis prius lotis nos venam rescindere."

of the Sultan's ill health. This expression calls to mind his earlier remarks on "the black bile arising from the combustion of phlegm" (136r, 8). "Combustion of the phlegm" appears to denote what would today be called "catarrh": a dripping downwards of fluid, as in the case of inflammation of the mucous membranes of the nose. In this way a pathophysiological basis to the author's system of medicine is revealed through a few remarks scattered throughout the instructions which he gives to a particular patient.

Chapter 16 is not found in the Jerusalem Hebrew text, although it appears in the Berlin manuscript. It consists of only six lines, which deal with some herbal and mineral remedies. These "act through specific properties, by which I mean their specific form which is the whole of their essence," so that it is impossible to explain their effects "through their particulars alone," or, in modern parlance, on a pharmacological basis. Maimonides brings, as an example, the cardiac medicaments, consisting of "exhilarating potions and the electuary in which there is jacinth, emerald, gold, and silver." The subject is discussed at length in the manuscript work *Sefer ha-Nisyonoth* (The Book of Experiments), which is attributed to Rabbi Abraham ibn Ezra.

Chapter 17 deals with a general medical problem, the habituation of the body to drugs which then cease to act as a medicament "and they turn into nourishment or the like of nourishment" (143r, 10 ff.). The author attributes this idea to Galen. Maimonides gives as an example the use of oxtongue, which he so highly praises, "despite which the cause of the disease has not disappeared." He maintains that this is because the Sultan has continued its use too long.

The difference between a medicament and a nutrient is discussed at length by Galen in *De naturalibus facultatibus*, Book III, 7 (K. II: 161) and in *De simplicium medicamentorum temperamentis*, III and V (K. XI: 545 and 705) and elsewhere. However, we could not find any mention of the question of habituation in the form in which Maimonides speaks of it. The idea of the transition of medicaments to nutriments is also to be found in Persian and Indian medicine. (See the tenth-century work by Abū Mansūr Muwaffak, translated by Achundow, reprinted 1968, p. 140).

Chapter 18 starts with the advice that the Sultan reduce the frequency of coitus (143v, 4–6). The brevity of this section may be due to the fact that the subject had been extensively covered in the Arabic medical literature of the time, and Maimonides had himself devoted two special treatises to it, containing psychological observations and advice on suitable drugs and diet. Perhaps, too, a sense of modesty prevented him from enlarging on the subject when addressing the Sultan.

The chapter then continues with more detailed instructions about bathing, sleeping, and exercising. Bathing (in hot water) "should never be neglected either during paroxysms of fever or in remissions" (143v, 7–8). Coitus and bathing are considered from a general point of view, while the other two subjects are dealt with mainly in connection with the condition of the Sultan. The author notes that his patient sleeps well and adds a theoretical comment to the effect that, although the "black vapors" affect the heart, they "do not hurt the brain or alter its temperament" (143v, 10–11). He thus links sleep with the state of the brain, a connection which has only been demonstrated in recent times. The problem of a "sleep-center" in the midbrain has been discussed by Kleitman in his very informative work *Sleep and Wakefulness*, 1939; in cases of sleep disorders, Mauthner (1890) found lesions localized in the periventricular grey, and v. Economo in the floor of the third ventricle (1923 to 1929). The title of Kleitman's work is perhaps an allusion to the Pseudo-Aristotelian treatise *De somno et vigilio*. For earlier references, Kleitman mentions the work of Piéron.

The chapter ends with the advice that the "weakness after exercise" of which the Sultan complains can be overcome by the gradual resumption of activity—in other words, by "training." Recent physiological investigations have shown that a healthy man who is not accustomed to exercise reacts to severe exertion in the same way as one who suffers from heart disease: that is, with an increased oxygen requirement. Maimonides deals with exercise at greater length in Section XVIII of his *Aphorisms*, where the ideas expressed are somewhat similar to those found in Galen's *De sanitate tuenda*, Book II, 2 (K. VI: 83 ff.).

Maimonides begins Chapter 19 by noting that he has now answered all the questions addressed to him in the "noble letter" of the Sultan. This is possibly the reason why the Florence incunable of the Latin version of the treatise ends with the eighteenth chapter. However, the Friedenwald and Vienna Latin manuscripts continue to the end of the original text.

The author states that in this chapter he will outline a general regimen for the Sultan. He admits that the bulk of these instructions is already to be found in the preceding part of this treatise, as well as in the *Regimen of Health*, "but these were statements that were dispersed and not properly organized" (144r, 15). He is thus following the principle given in the introduction to his theological Code (*Mishneh Torah*), where he states that his intention in that work is to bring together the whole of the oral law. However, here he precedes his instructions with a short prescription for a cardiac "electuary" taken, as he says, from a book of Rhazes, followed by a long prescription from Avicenna's work *De viribus cordis*. These were apparently so important to Maimonides that he hastened to give them before his general directions.

In Chapter 20 Maimonides suggests that, in addition to the medicaments mentioned in Chapter III of the *Regimen of Health*, both these electuaries should be prepared "in the treasury of our Master" (144v, 2)—that is, in the royal pharmacy—and kept there in case of need. This idea is also found in the introduction to his *Book of Poisons*, where he deplores the impossibility in Egypt of finding the herbs required to prepare theriac for the treatment of animal bites. Presumably for similar considerations, he here gives the prescriptions in full.

The somewhat complicated prescription attributed to Rhazes is said to have been taken from his treatise entitled *On the Repulsion of the Harm of the Nutrients*. According to Brockelmann, a manuscript of the Latin translation of this work exists in the Escurial Library, and an Arabic version is in Cairo. Again the subject of this book recalls Galen's discussion in *Ad Pisonem de theriaca*, Chapter 4 (K. XIV: 299) about the action of nutriments as drugs and the biological differences between the two (see our summaries of Chapters 17 and 20). This prescription does not contain oxtongue, a medicament which has already been discussed. It consists mainly of pleasant aromatics, some of them rare, which probably exert a stimulatory effect which is more psychological than pharmacological. Some of the ingredients of this prescription are also constituents of Avicenna's electuary, including citron leaves (154v, 12–15), which are recommended by him as a household remedy.

The mixture was supposed to be "an excellent medicament for strengthening the heart" (145r, 6–7), particularly in the case of "syncope" and of "throbbing of the heart." Neither of these conditions can be precisely defined and Arabic dictionaries provide various translations for the terms given. In medieval and Renaissance Latin, the name "lipothymia" was used to indicate an attack verging on, but less extreme than, collapse.

The second cardiac medicament is known as the "jacinth (ruby) electuary." It is identical with that given in *De viribus cordis* of Avicenna. This is the only place in his medical writings that Maimonides cites at length and word for word from another medical authority. The ingredients vary according to whether the final preparation is to be "cold" or "hot" or "temperate." Avicenna claims that he has added to and taken from this complicated prescription "according to each and every temperament" (145r, 16–17) of the patient. "Gold filings" and precious stones were added on magical grounds, as was also usual in the West in the Middle Ages and the Renaissance. Gold as a remedy was especially popular in the form of a drink, known as Aurum Potabile. In modern medicine the pure metal is not used, but the salts are injected for the treatment of arthritis (chrysotherapy).

The basic prescription seems to have been designed for a patient with a "moderate temperament" (145r, 9 to 146r, 16). This could be prepared in two forms, "as an electuary or in troches." There follow the modifications required for a hot temperament (146v, 1–9) and for a cold temperament (147r, 3–8), as well as for those with a hot temperament who are suffering from various cardiac complaints (147r, 8 to 148r, 14).

Opium, which first makes its appearance in the treatise on 146r, 12, is one of the few constituents which is known to exert a powerful pharmacological action.[3] However, it appears to have been used here, together with powdered castoreum, to cause the mixture to ferment. If that is done, the mixture should not be used for at

---

[3]   Most of the Arabic manuscripts clearly mention opium here (146r, 12), but MS. Paris refers to epithymum, as do the Latin versions.

least six months. Galen deals with the somniferous properties of opium in his book *De compositione medicamentorum secundum locos*, Book I, Chapter 4 (K. XIII: 274) and mentions the addition of hyoscyamus to produce "stupor," but he does not refer to fermentation. Nor does Muwaffak, who speaks of the use of opium against pain (Muwaffak, 1968, p. 170), as well as of opium poisoning, noting the lethal dose (pp. 165 and 179). However, the matter is discussed by William Heberden in his *Antitheriaca* (1745). Heberden, who in the spirit of his time opposed the use of theriac, brings as an argument the fact that the opium in it is likely to ferment and become still stronger and thus more harmful.[4]

In the prescription "for one who is dominated by a bad hot temperament" (146*r*, 10), epithymum was to be omitted, because it was thought to possess heating properties; certain "cooling" herbs were added, but "the other ingredients should be kept as they are" (146*v*, 7). The details of the cooling plants given in our Hebrew manuscript are somewhat abbreviated compared with Avicenna's original text.

Another amended prescription is for "those who follow the same course as kings suffering from melancholia" (147*r*, 4), that is, from the manic-depressive syndrome. At first it seemed to us that the disease was associated with the word "kings" because of its importance. Thus Celsus used the word "royal" in his description of jaundice: "morbus quem interdum regium nominant" (royal disease; *De medicina*, Book III, 24; p. 339 in Loeb Classical Library). However, we have discarded this interpretation of melancholy as a "royal disease" on medico-historical and textual grounds. The word "kings" appears to have been introduced by the author in order to appease the patient, thereby indicating that his condition is not uncommon and also affects persons of high rank (see our commentary on 147*r*, 4). For the treatment of melancholia, the author augments the action of the electuary with the addition of thoroughly powdered jacinth (ruby) (147*r*, 6). It is difficult to discover the possible pharmacological action of such substances in the light of modern medicine. (See our discussion above of the fact that minerals such as gold were regarded as acting through their "specific properties" rather than on pharmacological grounds).

Next follows the version for those with a hot temperament who suffer from "weakness of the heart" (147*r*, 8 ff.). This prescription is extremely detailed, containing numerous additions to the basic recipe; the additions are included because of qualities they were said to possess with reference to the humoral theory. Thus, for example, watermelon was thought to be "cooling and moistening to the second degree," so that it was prescribed by Avicenna and Maimonides for those cardiac symptoms which were believed to be due to a hot temperament (147*r*, 11). Precious

---

4 See Gilbert Watson, *Theriac and Mithridatium*, 1966, p. 139; "He (Heberden) recalls that theriac, according to Galen, was kept for a long time in order to mitigate the strength of the opium. This practice still persists, but the mixture is apt to ferment, the fermentation makes the opium three or four times stronger, and the mixture thus becomes much more dangerous."

stones and shredded silk were also added. The herbs prescribed were mainly aromatic stimulants for the treatment of "syncope," that is, loss of consciousness due to cardiac or circulatory conditions. These were strong-smelling substances, such as rosewater, saffron, or camphor, or else the juice of certain fruits such as quinces or apples. Oxtongue was also used for this purpose (147v, 11).

A "julep" is recommended (147v, 15 to 148r, 14) as a drink which "is beneficial to all those who have a weakness of the heart" (148r, 8–9). "Tabarzad sugar" is prescribed (148r, 3–4), apparently with the idea that carbohydrates are of value for such cases. Here too it is suggested that oxtongue might be added (148r, 9 and 13–14), showing that the opinion was prevalent that cardiac conditions were influenced by the state of mind. However, Maimonides also appears to have been aware that a disease process can also affect the heart substance (see Section III of his *Aphorisms*, Muntner's Hebrew edition, p. 40, § 14). The prescription ends with quantitative instructions regarding the drugs to be taken, according to "the temperament" of the patient.

Following this long quotation from Avicenna, Maimonides offers some succinct advice concerning the diet. He first deals with the preparation of bread, stating that it is not desirable to use flour that has been "made white." However, it cannot be claimed from this that he knew of the properties of the high-extraction loaf. Other details regarding the preparation of bread are to be found in the first chapter of his *Regimen of Health*, where he states: "The bread should be made of a coarse flour, that is to say that the husk should not be removed and the bran should not be refined by sifting." In our work however, he insists that "it should be sifted thoroughly until none of the bran remain in it" (148v, 4–5 and our running commentary to this passage). Apparently he had learned from Galen or Hippocrates that coarse bread exerts a laxative effect and is less nutritious.[5]

Maimonides speaks of the technical processes involved in the preparation of bread: steeping in water, winnowing, thorough kneading, the addition of salt, and adequate baking so that the heat penetrates well inside the loaf. He also discusses the type of oven to be used. It should be noted that bread is the first foodstuff to which Maimonides refers, since it was the staple food of the people but was also served at the table of kings.

Our author then deals with meat as food. He prefers birds, particularly "hens or roosters . . . because this sort of fowl has virtue in rectifying corrupted humors, . . . and especially the black humors" (atrabilis) (148v, 12–15). He gives detailed instructions about the care of these birds, mentioning the cleanliness of the runs, the content of the different feeds throughout the day (which are to include milk and

---

[5]   See Galen, *De alimentorum facultatibus* I, 2 (K. VI: 484) and elsewhere and also Mielck (1914). See also: Hippocrates, *Regimen*, II: 42, on the wheat for bread: "When cleaned from the bran it nourishes more, but is less laxative" (Jones edition, IV: 311).

dried figs), and the quantities of food to be provided (which should not be excessive) (149r, 15). In this way, "we find the suet white and delicious; it cooks as rapidly as possible, moistens the temperament greatly," and so on (149v, 6–7). If repetition of this diet becomes tedious, the Sultan may also occasionally take francolin, grouse, or turtledove, although these are drying.[6] Like Ibn Rushd (See Paulus Aegineta, Adams edition, I: 141), Maimonides does not recommend the partridge, because he believes it causes constipation.

He then proceeds to animal meat (149v, 15–16), "if the spirit craves the meat of cattle." Even so he prefers to recommend the meat of a suckling kid. Only if it be unavoidable does he sanction the meat of sheep (150r, 1), and then only "those lambs that have not attained a year." The meat "should not be excessively fat" and should be taken from grazing animals. His opposition to the meat of cattle is probably based on the idea, also mentioned by Galen, that the latter is not easily digested. Similar opinions about food are found in the Code (Hilkot de'ot, 4) of Maimonides, where he prescribes a strict diet even for healthy people.

Then follows a short section (150r, 6–14) on the subject of wine, which is recommended by Maimonides, despite the fact that it is proscribed to Muslims. In the subsequent section, it is also suggested that wine be added to a dish of chicken or meat. The author prefers white wine and objects to "that which is intensely red[7] or thick of essence . . . or old and intensely bitter," although slight astringency is not contraindicated.[8]

The author then discusses various dishes and shows a proficiency in those gastronomic matters which may be of concern to a prince. As to the medical implications, he adds: "Our master already knows the virtues of most of the foods" (150v, 2) and "a physician will not fail to be at hand to be relied on in this regard." Here again he prefers the meat of cocks or hens, for which he describes four methods of preparation: boiling, broiling, steaming, and cooking with herbs. He first lists the condiments and other substances to be used. Chervil (Anthriscus cerefolium) should be added in winter, lemon or citron in summer. Dishes prepared with currants,

---

6 See Hippocrates, De diaeta II: 47, and elsewhere. Ibn Zuhr, in the chapter on the types of meat in his De nutrimentis (Hebrew MS. Munich 220), also speaks of turtledoves and pigeons, describing their properties as heating and drying, while baby chicks "have the property of assuaging the type of headache known as migraine." This last statement may be compared with that of Maimonides concerning the turtledove, which "has a unique virtue in kindling the mind" (149v, 12).

7 With regard to color, Ibn Zuhr (in De nutrimentis, see above, p. 22, note 1) states that the sight of certain colors affects the body: looking at red things results in bleeding, and the sight of saffron-colored objects brings on jaundice.

8 About wine see Galen, Die säfteverdünnende Diät, Trans. Beintker & Kahlenberg, IV, p. 138: "thick wine which is also black and sweet fills the vessels with thick blood, while white and thin wines disperse the thick humors and purify the blood via the urine," and so on.

almonds, and a little vinegar "are excellent at any time." Nor should one neglect the addition of spices "to prevent any harm to the stomach" (151r, 2), a warning which has already been given a number of times.

The author then deals with the preparation of animal meat, which he suggests should be suckling kid, roasted on a spit. He advises that saffron be added "because it is a cheering cardiac medicament" (again the preoccupation with cardiac drugs), although too much should not be used, because it takes away the appetite (151v, 8).

The chapter ends with a discussion on hydromel and oxymel, which were so highly recommended by both Hippocrates and Galen. The first preparation was a mixture of water or thin white wine and honey, and the second consisted of vinegar and honey. Here Maimonides states that Galen's successors used sugar instead of honey in both cases. This changeover from honey to sugar is also discussed at length by Ibn Zuhr, who notes that sugar was more costly than honey and was used only by the royal house. Maimonides considers hydromel to be a most valuable drink (152r, 2–6) for "strengthening the stomach and the heart, improving the digestion, dilating the spirit," as well as for "easing the egress of the superfluities," that is, the stools and the urine, and he stresses: "We have tested it . . . time and again" (152r, 5–6).

As with his other recommendations, Maimonides provides quantitative directions for the preparation of hydromel, with indications as to when it should be taken and its effect on the temperament (152r, 1 to 152v, 7). At the end of this chapter, he again discusses the medical and nutritive properties of the substances to which he refers. The rule was that, whenever possible, nutrient substances should be used, rather than drugs. He cites as an example the use of sugar and wine, which were essentially nutrients in his opinion, although he believed that they possessed some medicinal qualities. (See our summary above of Chapter 17, where references to parallels in Galen's works are given, particularly in *De naturalibus facultatibus*.)

Chapter 21 concerns the regimen to be followed by the Sultan, with reference to the season of the year, eating habits, exercise, sleep, and so on. In his suggestions about exercise before meals, the author notes the following physiological criteria: warming of the limbs (153r, 8), changes in respiration, and sweating (lines 9–10). Following breakfast, sleep is recommended, to be induced by a singer accompanied by a stringed instrument "until he sleeps deeply" (153v, 4). This unusual time for sleep may be due to the fact that the Sultan was supposed to get up early, "at sunrise or a little before that" (153r, 2–3).

The idea of the soothing influence of music and its effect on sleep is attributed to the "physicians and philosophers" (153v, 5) — presumably a reference to the school of Pythagoras. Such psychological considerations (which include the question of suitable company) are intended to "dilate the psyche and remove evil thoughts from it" (153v, 14–15).

Before supper the Sultan was to take hydromel prepared with wine and also containing water of oxtongue (154r, 1). He was to wait half an hour before eating, until the beverage had left the stomach. This instruction was probably based on empirical findings, and indeed, drinking dilutes the stomach juices which are required to digest the meal. The drink was to be taken not only on account of its medicinal properties; the increased water requirements of the body in hot countries appear also to have been taken into account: "For it will be good and moistening to the body" (154r, 2–3). The author suggests that it would be best if the drink were to replace the evening meal, either entirely or with the sole addition of some condiment or of "citron peel preserved in sugar" which, he later stresses (154v, 13), does not "heat the temperament." However, if supper is taken (154v, 8), the instructions are repeated regarding the way in which the chickens for the meal should be fed and then cooked.

Following 154v, two pages are missing in the Jerusalem Hebrew MS. Here the Arabic original deals with the bath and also contains special dietary instructions concerning bathing. The author quotes Galen as saying that sleep is necessary after the bath, adding that supper should be omitted on that day.

The question of coitus is taken up again on 155r.[9] It should take place "neither during hunger upon an empty stomach nor when the stomach is filled with food" (155r, 4–5).[10] The same rules apply to drinking the "mixed [hydromel-oxtongue] drink" described above, and this gives the author the opportunity to repeat his dietetic theories in this regard (155r, 6). Drinking before the food in the stomach has been digested "will unripen it [the food] and expel it before its ripening."

At the end of the section on the general regimen for winter, there are further instructions concerning the time when Avicenna's prescriptions should be taken (155r, 12 to 155v, 3). This was considered to be a most important part of the regimen. On this same day (Friday) the Sultan was to refrain from exercise (155r, 13–14), and none of the medicaments taken were to contain castoreum (155r, 17), which was believed to act as a stimulant (see Meyerhof, 1940, no. 79).

Instructions with regard to the regimen in the hot season begin on 155v, 3. The Sultan was to be awakened from sleep an hour after daylight. This was later than in winter, presumably on account of the length of the day, though he would still be able to benefit from the coolness of the air. He was to take only very little of the "mixed drink," but "the cool musk medicament" and "the cool jacinth medicament" (see 145r, 12) are recommended. It has previously been noted that musk was supposed to have the property of "strengthening the heart" (141r, 1; 147v, 9); this was one of the constituents of the formula of Ibn Sīnā's cardiac remedy intended for those suffering from a "bad, hot temperament" together with cardiac manifestations, such as "palpitation and weakness of the heart" (147r, 9–11).

---

9   See the short sections on reducing the frequency of coitus on 142v, 4–6 and on 155b, 11.

10 See Galen *De constitutione artis medicae*, Chapter 24, (K. I: 372): "Nempe immodicae repletionis et inanitionis."

The author then discusses the drink to be taken after the bath (156r, 1), the laxative to be given if required, and the addition of barley porridge or gruel (*kashk*) if the weather gets hotter, with the proviso that at night it should be taken "instead of foods and drinks that fill the stomach"(156r, 11–12). Barley water is prescribed by Maimonides in his *Aphorisms* (Muntner Hebrew edition, p. 245) "to thin the thick humors." Its use in stomach conditions is dealt with in detail by Ibn al-Bayṭar (Sontheimer, II: 97).

In the present work, Maimonides speaks of barley porridge (156r, 6 to 156v, 9), to be made of polished barley with the addition of fumitory, endive, oxtongue, poppy seed, sandalwood, nard, dill and olive oil. This mixture was to be cooked over a charcoal fire until half the water had evaporated. Wine vinegar was then added and the heating continued until less than a quarter remained (156v, 7). Ibn al-Bayṭar (Sontheimer, II: 97) cites a similar recipe in the name of Galen. Maimonides credits this preparation with the following properties: "It will resist the dryness of the black humor, moderate the inflamed humors, remove their burnings, thicken those vapors that ascend to the heart and the brain, prevent their ascent, cool the temperament through moderation" (156v, 12 ff.).

Maimonides apparently follows Hippocrates in his enthusiasm for medicinal barley preparations. He is also aware of the side effects of the substances added to the mixture, including those of opium, which should not be taken if "there is constipation or acidity in the stomach" (that is, hyperacidity). Here the Jerusalem Hebrew manuscript ends with the words: "Hippocrates says . . ." The last three pages of the original text are thus lacking here, but they are to be found in the three Latin manuscripts which we have examined.

In the Arabic text the discussion on the virtues of barley porridge is then continued. In the *Regimen*, Book II (Jones edition, IV: 309 ff.), Hippocrates speaks at length of barley cakes and a barley drink. He also refers to barley porridge (gruel) throughout his *Regimen in Acute Diseases* and many of his indications are found in our text.

The next chapter, which is numbered 22 in the Kroner edition, is the last of the treatise. It seems that Maimonides was feeling too weak and ill to appear in person before the Sultan and therefore gave his answer in writing. He does not bemoan his state, but in the spirit of the Talmudic phrase (*Berakot*, 40b) thanks the Almighty equally for his good and bad fortune. It is possible that he mentions his own frailty on psychological grounds, in order to remind the Sultan that perfect health is unattainable for most people.

Maimonides then justifies his recommendation of wine and song, which are generally forbidden to Muslims: "The physician, because he is a physician, must give information on the conduct of a beneficial regimen, be it unlawful or permissible, and the sick have the option to act or not to act." It should be noted that in his *Aphorisms*, which were addressed to Jews as well as to non-Jews, Maimonides himself speaks of "eating the head of a hare" (Section 22), a food which is forbidden by Jewish law, although it is true that he cites this whole section in the name of the Muslim physician Ibn Zuhr. In the present treatise Maimonides even adds that "if the physician refrains from prescribing all that is of benefit, whether it be prohibited or permissible [according to religious law] he deceives, and does not deliver his true counsel." Thus he distinguishes between religion and medicine. "The Law [religion] commands whatever is of benefit and prohibits whatever is harmful in the next world, while the physician gives information about what is beneficial to the body and warns against whatever harms it in this world," In any case the prescription of wine for a believing Muslim ruler would appear to be an act of courage on the part of Maimonides. Incidentally, in the Hebrew translation of Ibn Zuhr's treatise on diet, which is quoted in our text, there is no word about wine in the long passage on beverages, possibly on religious grounds. However, the use of wine is discussed by Avicenna in his *Canon* (Venice edition, 1593, I: 180).

A detailed discussion on the passages dealing with the subject of medicine and religion, with which Maimonides closes his treatise, is given at the end of our running commentary.

A PALAEOGRAPHIC DESCRIPTION
OF THE JERUSALEM HEBREW MANUSCRIPT

M. BEIT-ARIÉ

INTRODUCTION

MANUSCRIPT Heb. 8⁰ 3941 of the Jewish National and University Library in Jerusalem, which contains the text of this critical edition, is very interesting from a palaeographic point of view and offers a challenge to the palaeographer. It presents a few unusual features, some of them hitherto unknown to us.

The importance of detailed and comprehensive palaeographic description and analysis in the critical edition of a manuscript is well known. Textual and critical problems may be solved by such study. Palaeographic and codicologic description sheds light on the history of the text of the manuscript and its transmission and provides the textual critics with information on the differentiation of hands, glosses and corrections, missing pages, and other archaeological aspects.

The manuscript considered here is part of a collection of more than one hundred manuscripts belonging to Rabbi Ḥayyim Beḵor (Gilibi) ben Ephraim ha-Levi (HiBaH). The collection was bought by the Library in 1962 from the grandson of HiBaH in Jerusalem. Rabbi Ḥayyim Beḵor ha-Levi was born in Ismir in 1815 and died there in 1908. His ancestors, who had been expelled from Spain, settled in Venice and later moved to Constantinople. He himself lived in Constantinople for a time. There he practiced medicine, including the methods used in the practical Kabbala, for which he earned a wide reputation. He was well-known as the private physician of the mother of the Sultan 'Abd al-'Azīz (M. D. Gaon, 1938, p. 730). It is therefore not surprising that his collection includes a considerable number of medical manuscripts.

The complete manuscript 8⁰ 3941 consists of six works, written by three different hands. It can be divided into three bibliographic units, which coincide with the three palaeographic units, as follows:

1. Fol. 1r–13v: An essay on resurrection by Maimonides, known in the Hebrew translation of Samuel Ibn Tibbon as *Ma'amar Tĕḥiyyat haMetim*. The translator is unknown.

2. Fol. 14v–19v: A copy of a hitherto unknown commentary of the Tractate *Avot* of the *Mishna*, in a different script.

3. Fol. 20r–156v: The main part of the manuscript, consisting of four medical works by Maimonides, written in still another script, in a previously unknown Hebrew translation. (For a detailed description, see Beit-Arié, 1962–1963). The last of these is the text studied in this volume (130v–156v). The others are briefly:

34

a) Fol. 20r–78v: A translation of *Maqāla fī'r-Rabw* (*Treatise on Asthma*). The translation differs from both the popular translation of Samuel Benveniste (edited by Muntner, 1940) and the lesser known translation of Joshua Shatibi (Steinschneider, 1875, no. 280).

b) Fol. 79r–84v: A translation of *Fī'l Jimā'* (*On coitus*), shorter version. The translation in our manuscript differs from the two known versions.[1]

c) Fol. 84r–130v: מאמר שמירת הבריאות, a translation of *Fī tadbīr aṣ-ṣiḥḥat*, which differs from the known translation of Moses Ibn Tibbon. (For bibliographical details, see Beit-Arié, p. 568.)

The four medical works were written by the same hand and thus belong to the same palaeographic unit. It can be assumed from the style in which they are written that all are from the same translator. The fact that the four works are grouped together as a corpus may shed some light on the mode of transmission of the texts; the medical works of Maimonides are frequently found grouped together in a particular order in Arabic sources, as well as in Hebrew and Latin translations.

The three palaeographic units of the manuscript differ in the morphology of the letters, as well as in such graphic and technical features as completion of the line, methods of writing words in the margin, catchwords, abbreviation signs, and substitutions for the tetragram. Even so, there are elements in common which allow us to consider the whole manuscript as one, rather than three, palaeographic units. The main features in common are the special composition of the quires, the writing material, and the ruling. The standard system of numbering the quires, to be discussed later, provides strong evidence that the entire manuscript was copied by three scribes in the same place and during the same period of time. There is a great affinity between the script of the second part and that of the main section, the former appearing to be a cursive variant of the latter. The third part starts with a new quire, but the second part begins in the middle of a quire. One can conclude from this that there is a direct connection between the first two parts.

The script of the main manuscript, which includes our text, is impressive. It is semisquare and unusually large in size. But it also contains primitive elements, such as the system used for ruling, the variable number of lines, and the nonuniform layout. It is difficult to establish a location for this type of script. It includes Sephardic, Italian, and oriental elements and also bears an affinity to Karaite writing. There are features typical of the Byzantine type of Hebrew script, and it is very likely that the manuscript was in fact written in Greece. This hypothesis is supported by the system of numbering the quires: at the head of each quire we find the numbering in Greek letters. This is the first time we have seen such a system in a Hebrew manuscript. The scarcity of Hebrew manuscripts written in Byzantium makes it difficult

---

[1] These two translations have been published, together with the long version of the original, by Kroner, 1906.

to date the manuscript. A morphological comparison was made with the other manuscripts written in Byzantium, such as MS. Paris héb. 177, written in 1308, MS. Oxford Opp. Add. 4to 160, fol. 13–164 (Neubauer, 1886–1906, no. 2518), written in Thebes in 1367,[2] and MS. New York Jewish Theological Seminary L827, written in Magnesia (western Turkey) in 1387, the scripts of which are more like the first in our manuscript and the heading scripts of which resemble that of our main manuscript. A morphological comparison was also made with later manuscripts, such as Oxford Mich. 261 (Catalogue no. 203), written in 1429; Oxford Opp. Add. 4to 28 (Catalogue no. 1095), written in Rhodes in 1426 and Paris héb. 237, written in Kastoria (Macedonia) in 1437. From this and from other features, such as the type of paper used, it may be assumed that our manuscript was written in or near Greece at the end of the thirteenth century.

DETAILED DESCRIPTION

1. *Material:* The manuscript is written on paper and parchment; the parchment is reserved for the outer and inner sheets of each quire. The paper is very thick and stout. It has a glossy surface and is brownish in color. The pulp is irregular, the laid and chain lines are hardly visible, and there are no watermarks. The space between the chain lines is 50–59 millimeters. The width of every 20 laid lines is 43–45 millimeters. The laid lines are not parallel but vertical to the written lines, thus indicating that the original format of the sheet was *quarto* and its size (according to the actual trimmed size) was 430 millimeters by 300 millimeters. These features correspond to the early prewatermark occidental papers,[3] especially to the Italian paper found in dated Greek manuscripts of the second half of the thirteenth century. The morphology of the chain lines and the format of our manuscript resemble MS. Parisinus Gr. 618, dated 1298, and the morphology of the laid lines and the size of the sheet is similar to MS. Parisinus Gr. 2207, dated 1299.[4]

The parchment is of medium thickness and is perhaps made of goat skin. It is possible to distinguish between its sides; the hair side is only crudely shaved, if at all. The text is written in brown ink.

2. *Quires:* Each quire has six sheets (twelve leaves),[5] four of paper and two, the

---

2 Compare the facsimile of this manuscript in Neubauer, Facsimiles, 1886, Pl. XXIV. The date 1267, which is given in the colophon, is reproduced in both the album and the catalogue. However, this must be corrected, because it appears that the hundreds (one hundred years) were omitted by mistake from the Hebrew date, as is proved by the appearance of the watermarks and by chronological examination.

3 Cf. the detailed description by Irigoin, 1950, especially pp. 197–198 and 202. See also Irigoin, 1953.

4 Irigoin, 1950, p. 197.

5 This kind of composition is found in many Hebrew manuscripts written in Spain, Provence, and North Africa (the domain of Sephardic culture) from the end of the thirteenth century on, but only in Greece and its surroundings does it represent the most usual size of the quire.

outer and the inner sheets, of parchment. In all the quires, the hairside of the outer sheet and the fleshside of the inner sheet are to the outside, except for quires nos. 4 and 6, in which the hairside is outside on both the outer and inner sheets. The technique of paper-parchment quires is found in Hebrew manuscripts written in Spain, Italy, and Byzantium.[6] The earliest dated Hebrew manuscript using this technique hitherto known to me is one of Spanish origin, written in 1225.[7] The technique is also found in the Hebrew manuscripts written in Italy from the fourteenth century on, but it was very common in Hebrew manuscripts written in Greece, Crete, Rhodes, and Northern Byzantium in the fourteenth and fifteenth centuries.[8]

Catchwords, most of which are decorated in a simple fashion, appear at the end of the quires, and signatures of Greek letters are found at the beginning of each quire. In the quires of the first and second hands, there are also catchwords at the end of each folio.[9]

Lacunae: The following pages are missing: the first quire and three pages of the second; the first page (parchment) of the fourth quire (after fol. 19); the ninth quire (after fol. 78, which contained the end of the *Treatise on Asthma* and the beginning of *On Coitus;* one page after fol. 154; and four pages at the end of the last quire. The interior parchment sheet of the third quire includes one stub.

3. *Ruling:* The manuscript was ruled in an unusual way. Only frames were drawn, and these very crudely by drypoint. No lines were ruled, and indeed the number of the lines is not even identical on both sides of the same folio. No traces of pricking are visible. In general, the folios of each half-folded quire were ruled together from the recto of the upper parchment folio. Since the paper is very thick, the ruling is distinct only in the first folios. Sometimes the parchment folios were ruled separately, and a few of the parchment folios at the beginning of the second half of the folded quire were not ruled at all; there are no traces of ruling in any of the folios of the second half of the quire.

4. *Disposition:* The total size of the paper is 214 millimeters by 145 to 146 millimeters. The text size is 130 to 145 millimeters by 85 to 100 millimeters. The number of lines on each page varies from 16 to 23 and the length of the written lines from 58 to 77 millimeters.

---

6   Cf. Beit-Arié, 1969–1970, p. 438.

7   Jerusalem, Jewish National and University Library, Yah. MS. Heb. 1, in which the outer sheet of each quire is made of parchment. The same technique is found in one of the earliest Latin manuscripts written on occidental paper (manufactured in Spain), MS. Paris, Bibliothèque Nationale, nouvelles acquisitions 1296, from the second half of the twelfth century (cf. Irigoin, 1950, p. 200).

8   Concerning such a technique in Byzantine Greek manuscripts see Irigoin, 1950, p. 221.

9   The earliest dated Hebrew manuscript hitherto known to me in which there are catchwords at the end of the folios is MS. Oxford Hunt. 164 (catalogue no. 1249), written in Mardin (Iraq) in 1292. However, catchwords are already found at the end of the folios of the first half of the quire in MS. Jerusalem (see n. 7) from Spain, dated 1225.

5. *Boundaries:* Lines are completed by elongation of letters and by graphic line endings. Protruding letters are written above the end of the line, protruding words are written obliquely downwards.

6. *Vocalization:* Occasional vocalization appears for ambiguous words. The *qames* and *patah* are not differentiated, in accordance with the so-called Sephardic pronunciation.

7. *Decoration:* Headings are written in large square letters.

8. *Corrections and marginalia:* Alternate readings, written in the margin by the scribe, refer to words indicated by three dots in the form of a triangle. In the first medical work only (*Treatise on Asthma:* fol. 20r–78v), equivalent terms in Latin and in an unidentified dialect (perhaps Greek) are indicated in the same manner. Cancellation is indicated by short oblique lines above the word. A change in the order of words or letters is indicated by placing one dot above the word or letter to be read first and two dots above that to be read next. The separation of contracted words is designated by two vertical dots. A number of marginal notes by later hands have been written in Greek script, and others are in late Sephardic script, probably from Turkey.

CONCLUSIONS

The text studied in this book is part of a Hebrew manuscript written in Byzantium (Greece or its environs), probably at the end of the thirteenth century. The manuscript shows signs of formal calligraphy, but it also presents primitive features in its bookcraft techniques. It was probably copied for the personal use of the scribe.

From the alternate marginal readings added by the same hand, it would seem that the copyist collated at least two manuscripts for his version. It may also be assumed that he copied the integral version of one manuscript only and collated the alternate readings of another in the margin, without mixing the two versions.

מאמר ההכרעה
לר׳ משה בן מימון

The 13th Century Hebrew Translation of the Arabic Text,
reproduced in facsimile with annotations
and corrections

MOSES MAIMONIDES
ON THE CAUSES OF SYMPTOMS

The English Translation from the Arabic Original,
with a Running Commentary

אדונינו יתמיד לו הבריאותוי מעינו
יתֵ תכלית טובת השני עולמות כמו
שהמציא לעבדין ולאן הנכבדים
שבבריואין כחסדין ועובן וכבודו:

ומרשיתו

מאמר ההכרעה
הדירוי אחר
לרבי משה זעל

זה החסד
מן ספרי
הרופא

1

בשם האל הרחמן הרחום הא׳
הפך רצון ושלום:
בא אל העבד הקטון הכתב הכולל
חילוק אותם המקרים כולם שהיעו
לאדונינו יאריך האומין ובאר טבות
אותם המקרים כולם וזמע א׳

יתמיד

5

1: ‏החסד‎] In the margin. Should read ‏החסר‎.   8: ‏יאריך‎] In the margin ‏יתמיד‎.

Wherever the manuscript is difficult to read, the words in question are given without further annotation.

In these annotations, references to the Arabic source are given in accordance with the text published by Kroner (based on MSS. Cod. Uri 555 (Poc. 313) and Cod. Poc. 280 (Neubauer 1270[5])) and reproduced in this volume (pp. 165–188).

40

1

Another work,
The Treatise of Decision,
offered in a spirit of friendship,
by Rabbi Moses, may the memory
of the righteous be blessed *

This [treatise]
is missing
from the
works of
the physician*

In the name of God, the Merciful and the compassionate; God,
show Thy good will and grant reward*

5

A letter has reached this minor Servant containing a list of all those accidents that have befallen our Master, may God perpetuate his days, along with an explanation of the causes of all those accidents and the times

1–3 Maimonides gave no title to the work. Some of the manuscripts bear no title at all; others have been provided with a caption by the medieval translator or scribe (see our introduction, pp. 11–12). The Jerusalem manuscript is headed: "Another work, *The Treatise of Decision*, offered in a spirit of friendship, by Rabbi Moses of blessed memory." The allusion to friendship may imply that the author had no intention of hurting the feelings of his colleagues when he expressed divergent opinions. In the margin the scribe notes: "This is [the book] that was missing from the works of the physician [Maimonides]."

4–5 The first line of the invocation is in the form usually found in Arabic books from the Koran onward. In the Hebrew text, a phrase has been added which rhymes with the first line: "God, show Thy good will and grant reward."

---

* The title, invocation, and marginal note have been translated from the Hebrew text.

קיריתם ארעׄונם והספור בכל חלקיהן אׄ   1
שׁעריך הרופא לשאול בעבורם
וזכר מה שמתעהׂג כן בכל עת לכל
מקרה מהן וכתב בן מזה שיעצו
הרופאׄים בעשיתן ממה שהסליגו   5
עלין ונחלקו בן וידעהׄעבד הקטן
ידיעה אמתית שאותן הכתב מפי
אדונגן בלי ספק והׄעבדׄ נשבעׄא
יתעׄ שהמשובחים שׁ ברופׄאׄי דׄורגן
מק צריׄסׄ מׄידׄיעת הׄכרח מלאׄוׄי   10
אותה הקבׄיׄלה כל שבן שיפרׄשה
ומחברין אותה אותגן החיבור לפׄי
ראה העבד הקטן שתהׄיה שׄׄוכתו
לאדׄון עבדותגן ימׄמׄיד הׄל עלו אׄ
דברי רופא לה דברי רופא לׄמׄי שאׄל   15

(marginal notes: חיבור, מלאׄוׄי)

1: ארעונם] In the margin קרייתם.   4: מזה] Should read מה.   9: יתע] Abbreviation of יתעלה.
10: מלאוי] In the margin חיבור.   12: לפי] Abbreviation of לפיכך.   15: רופא] Following
this, the word לרופא, the equivalent of طبيب, is missing.   לה] Text corrected by a later
hand to לא.

1 of their occurrence, information on all the particulars that a physician
needs to inquire about, a description of his thoughts at each time about
5 each accident, and an outline of what the physicians advised and wherein
they agreed or disagreed. This minor Servant knows with certainty that
this letter was dictated by our Master, without a doubt. This Servant
swears by God the Most High, that accomplished physicians in our times
10 lack the knowledge essential for systematizing such complaints, let alone
explaining and organizing them in such a fashion. Therefore, this minor
Servant has seen to it that his answer to him who holds him in bondage,
15 may God preserve his shadow, is in the words of one physician to another
and not in the words of a physician to someone who is not

2 Maimonides states that he is in possession of the medical history of the
patient through a letter dictated by the Sultan. The fact that he opens the
treatise in this way shows that he appreciates the importance of history-
taking. The art of medical questioning was demonstrated by Hippocrates in
Prognostics, for example in the passage on the so-called facies hippocrat-
ica; Jones edition II: 9–10. There exists a special treatise by Rufus of
Ephesus on questions which a physician needs to ask. (See Daremberg and
Ruelle, 1879, pp. 195–215; Hans Gärtner, 1962.)

5–6 The consilium of doctors had given various opinions on which the author
was to comment.

8–12 in our times: The author censures the physicians of his time, thus implying
his reverence for the ancient authorities. In his *Treatise on Asthma*, XIII, he
does not refrain from criticizing those physicians who have not reached the
"boundary" (*gevul*), that is, the peak of knowledge in their field. (See the
Hebrew text, edited by S. Muntner, p. 38, line 23.)

10 systematizing: In the Hebrew version the word *ḥibbur* is given for the Arabic
naẓm which, among other meanings, denotes threading pearls on a string.
This may serve as a metaphor indicating that it is the practice of the physician to accumulate observations on which to base his conclusions.

14 shadow: Recalls the Biblical phrase "shall abide under the shadow of the
Almighty" (Psalm 91:1). The Arabic word has different meanings according
to the vocalization: in one, duration of life; in the other, shadow.

מאנשי המלאכה שכבר נתבאר לעבד
שלמות אדוננו בידיעת אותם המקדים
וסכותם וכבר ידע העבד אותם
המקריים הנחים עתה והם שאתדל
לריחותם · וכבר זכר אדוננו
לעבדו הקטן מה שיעץ כל רופא לוהו
שיזכור מה שאעל במאמר כל אחד
מהם וסר למשמעתנו : פרק

אמנם מאמר מי
שאמר מהרופאים שאן טא אדם מפיות
הגדים עתה כמו שכבר בא במקצת
העתים הין מסתלקין אותם המקריים
הנמצאים עתה הוא מאמר אמת
אין ספק בן והוא שאותן הדם שיבא
אינו כי אם עכירות הדם ושמריו

10: אדם] Should read הדם. Has been corrected in the text by the scribe.

1 of the people of the Art, since the perfection of our Master has become evident to this Servant through the account of those accidents and their causes.

Whereas this Servant is acquainted with those accidents that are now
5 present, the removal of which is desired, and whereas our Master, having cited to his minor Servant what each physician has counseled, has commanded him to comment on the statement of each one of them, he obeys accordingly:

10 As to the statement of the physicians who said that the ailments now   Chapter 1 present would disappear if the blood were to exude now from the orifices of the vessels as has already happened at times, it is the truth, without any
15 doubt. This is because that blood that comes out is only the turbidity of the blood and its sediment,

---

4   that are now present: The Arabic word also has the meaning of "being established" (Dozy). The Hebrew translation *nahim* connotes "being at rest" or "seated," which brings to mind the title of Morgagni's classical work on pathology, *De sedibus et causis morborum*, 1761.

11–12 as already happened at times: Here the physician notes the fact that these symptoms had previously occurred in the course of the disease.

11   In historical medicine, the terms vein, artery, ligament, and nerve were often used indiscriminately. See Lane, I, (1863–1893), Pt. 5, p. 2019; also Hyrtl, (1879), p. 194. Hence the differences between the Jerusalem and Berlin Hebrew manuscripts. See also: C. M. Goss (1961), a translation from Galen, K. III: 779–830.

15   The turbidity of the blood and its sediment: Clotted blood in the varicose veins. Similar ideas are expressed in Maimonides' treatise, *On Hemorrhoids*, Chapter 2: "When there is an excess of black bile in the blood, it becomes thick and turbid and is rejected by the organs; this turbid sediment descends to the lower part of the body and in this way the excrescences are produced and these are the hemorrhoids."

45

והטבע דוחהו לרוע שלו על דרך פאות 1

הבחירין · ואמנם מי שיעץ מהרופאו

בפתיחת הגידין כמילות ישב כהן

או לבדין ישב עליהן הוא חטא ואין

העבד רואה בזה בשום פנים מֵפְנֵי ~ 5

פעם רבים יבארוס העבד תחלתם

שאותם הדברים שסובלים אותם

מלמטה או ישב כדומיהם הֵם חַיִּים

ולפעמים יחממו המזג ושורפין

הלחות· והשני שאן הגידיס ~ 10

כשיפתחס הטבע פותח אותם בְּשִׁעוּר

מה שצריך וכשנפתחס אֵנֵ׳קֵרים

לפעמיס יפתחו ביתר מכ̇ו ̄

שלאוי ותֵיבה הגרת הדס ̇יֵתקשה

החזקתו ולפעמ׳ יארעזה כאשר יֵבֵֿא 15

1   expelled by Nature, because of its badness, in the form of a crisis. As for
the physician who advised opening the orifices of the vessels by means of
water in which one sits, or poultices on which one sits, he is in error. This
5   Servant does not agree with this at all, for several reasons which he will
explain. First, those things that are applied, or the hot water in which one
10   sits, heat the temperament and inflame the humors. Second, when Nature
opens these vessels, she opens them in the required measure, but when we
open them by medication, they open more than they should, the flow of
15   blood goes to excess and its arrest becomes difficult. Even when it comes

1   expelled by Nature, because of its badness: The elimination of pathological
matter, often designated as "residues" or "superfluities," is an ancient
biological idea, which is here applied to the bleeding from hemorrhoids.
(See also our commentary on 132*v*, 12). Galen (K. XVI: 133) advises venesection for this purpose when the bleeding is suppressed.

Maimonides, in his *Aphorisms*, Section 23, also speaks of a power of
expulsion which makes the superfluities descend to the "mouths of the
anal vessels." In the passage previously quoted from the treatise *On Hemorrhoids*, he comments on the rejection of the superfluities with the words: "the
organs are disgusted by them." Avicenna's views on the "superfluities" are
found in Book I of his *Canon* (Gruner's translation, p. 479).

2   crisis: Buḥrān; *see* Lane, I, Pt. 1, p. 157: "the crisis of a disease in change to
health, or to the contrary." In the Berlin manuscript the Hebrew translator
adds the words: "This is to say, the border" (*gevul*), meaning the end of the
phase of the disease.

9–10   heat the temperament and inflame the humors: A warning against the use
of treatments which may disturb the harmony of the humors and lead to
dyscrasia.

מעצמו עירבה עד שלא יוכל להרחיקן

והג שלו הגידין כשיפתחו מעצמן מה

שיבא מהן ברוב היו הדבר שראוי ~

לצאת מפני שדחה אותן הטבע לקצוות

והטבעה כח הדוחה לדחות אותן

וכשנפתחם אנחנו לפעמים יבא מה

שאין ראוי לצאת וכשיצא ממנו שום

דבר יהיה הבא ממנו ממה שראוי

לצאת יותר זה הכלל שאנחנו לא צריך

לזה הפועל אא כשיתנפחו אותם

המקנמות ויגדל כאבם מה נעשך

אז לפתיחתם בסמנין עד שיגר מה

שנדחה שם מהדם שנפח אותן ~

המקומות ויהיה פעלנ אז דומה

1 by itself, it may happen that it goes to excess so that it cannot be arrested.

Third, when these vessels open by themselves, whatever comes out of
them is most often what should come out, because Nature has driven it to
5 the periphery and the expulsive force has moved to expel it. If we open
them ourselves, something might come out that should not come out, and
most often this is what happens.

10 In general, we do not have recourse to this action unless those places
are swollen, and the pain is greatly increased. Then we open them by
medication so that whatever was dispelled there from the blood and caused
those places to swell flows out. Our action at such a time

12 open them by medication: The author does not specify his therapy. Hippocrates names several drugs, not in order to "open" the hemorrhoids but
presumably to exert an astringent effect (see Gurlt, I: 274). Generally Hippocrates is less conservative, and in his treatise *On Hemorrhoids* he first suggests
cutting the piles (Chapters 2,3) and only later mentions diet, poultices, and
so on. He considers the presence of hemorrhoids in certain diseases a favor-
able sign (*Aphorisms* VI, 11,12,21). Galen explains that spontaneous bleeding
from hemorrhoids is beneficial, because the *atra bilis* can thus be eliminated.
Only when the bleeding is suppressed should the hemorrhoids be incised
(*Hippoc. Epid. VI et Galeni in illum commentarius* V, Section 25, K. XVII
B: 286–287).

However, surgical treatment of hemorrhoids is clearly advised by Maimonides in his *Aphorisms* (XV): "The excrescence at the anus, the hemorrhoids,
must be cut."

נפֿח

דומה לפועל מי שפתח פוסתימא   1
שלא יכול הטבע לפתח מה שעל
הפוסתימא ולהוציא מה שיש בו ואין
ראוי שיעשה אדוננו זה בשום פנם ·
אבל אם נפתחו מעצמן כמו שאיך ע׳   5
פעמים אין ראוי להפסיקן בשום לא
אם הרבה חס ושלום: פרק
כפר זכר האדון שקצת הרופאים
יען בלקיחת מעט מהיין בלקיחת
מעט מהיין במי עשב לשון שור אחר   10
הכאכל בשעות ושיקח ממנו מעט
בעת השינה כדי שירדם בשינה
ושיקצתם יען בהפך זה ואמ אין שום
פנס לעשייתן שהחי ממנו מחמם
המזג ומוליד הרוחות למנפח ומה   15
שרואהן השמש שהגבעה הראשונה

1: דומה] Word repeated by mistake.   פוסתימא] In the margin נפח.   פוסתימא] Following this, the word באיזמיל is missing (found in MS Berlin).   6: בשום] Following this, פנים should be added (in MS Berlin צד).   9–10: בלקיחת מעט מהיין] Phrase repeated by mistake.   13: ואמ] Abbreviation of ואמר.   15: המזג] Following this, according to the Arabic والمزوج should read והמזוג יוליד, يولد.

50

1 is similar to the action of one who lances a swelling when Nature is unable to open that which overlies the swelling and expel what is in it. Our Master
5 should never do this, but, should it come by itself, as it has done several times, it should not be stopped at all, unless it goes to excess; may God avert it!

Our Master then mentioned that some of the physicians advocate taking   Chapter 2
13 a little wine with water of oxtongue a few hours after the meal and at bedtime to deepen his sleep, and that some of them advised in this regard that there is no purpose in its use, since the unmixed heats the temperament
15 and the mixed generates ventosity and flatus. As this Servant sees it, the first view

5–7 Although the author does not generally advocate the opening of hemorrhoids, he does not advise stopping spontaneous bleeding, unless the quantity of blood lost is excessive.

8 Here begins a long discussion of the use of "a little wine with water of ox-tongue" (*Buglossos*, or *Anchusa officinalis L.*, and several species of *Borraginaceae*). No contemporary pharmacological proof of the efficacy of this plant is known to us to have been published. However, preliminary results of investigations kindly performed at our request were reported to us in June of 1970: A crude extract from the root bark of *Anchusa italica* exerts a tranquilizing effect in animals (R. Mechoulam, Hebrew University, Jerusalem and H. Ederi, Tel Aviv University). The plant was known as *Euphrosynum* in ancient medicine, because it was thought to promote a good mood (Pliny, 25, 8, 40, § 81).

The psychotropic action is also mentioned by Dioscorides IV: 126 [128]; Galen, *De simplicium medicamentorum*, Book VI, Chapter 2, § 12. (K. XI: 852); Ibn al-Bayṭār (II: 437 in Sontheimer's translation: very detailed references). Meyerhof (1940, no. 211) only mentions that the druggists in Egypt sell *Borrago officinalis*, under the name "oxtongue," as a sudorific and diuretic remedy. The uses of "a little wine with water of oxtongue" are enumerated in our treatise as follows: (1) promoting sleep (133*r*, 12); (2) assisting digestion (133*v*, 3–4); and (3) eliminating the superfluities via the urine, as well as the "vapors" from the blood (133*v*, 4–7). The special indication of "dilation of the spirit" is mentioned later (133*v*, 11–12).

היא האמתית והוא שהמעט ממנו והוא 1

אוקיה כנעניח אן קרובלה כשיתחיל

המאכל בעיכול מה שמסייע על

העיכול ומסייע על צאת היתרונות כהרקת

השתן ומרחיק מהדם האדים 5

העשנים המולידים לאן המקריס

הנמצאים עתה כולס וכל שכן

כשיין מזג כמי לשון שור וכשורין כן

לשון השור עצמו שיעור שע דרהם

כאוקיה יהיה יותר נמרץ ויהיה 10

הרחבת לנפש יותר וזה אמרותו

הרופאים שהמשקה המשמח

כמוחלט אינם רוצים בו כי אם

משקה לשון שור וכשיושם לשון השור

במשקה מעסיק כהרחבת הנפש 15

---

1 is the correct one; that is, if the food has begun to be digested, a little of it
namely a Syrian ounce or the like, will help digestion, aid the egress of the
5 superfluities by promoting a copious flow of urine, and expel from the
blood the smoky vapors engendering all these presently occurring accidents,
especially if mixed with water of oxtongue. Should oxtongue itself be
10 infused in it, in a measure of two drams per ounce, it will be most effective,
and its dilation of the spirit will be greater.

When the physicians speak of the drink that exhilarates, in general they
15 mean the syrup of oxtongue. If the oxtongue is steeped in wine, it increases
the dilation

1–6 An enumeration of the beneficial effects of the mixture. One of these is the
elimination of "superfluities" through the urine. This indicates some notion
of the function of "clearance" of the urine, an activity of the kidneys which
is measured in modern medicine. About "the nature of the superfluities,"
see Galen, *On the Natural Faculties*, translated by Brock, 1928, Book I, x,
pp. 35–37: "Nature, therefore, had need of a second process of separation
for the superfluities." See our introduction, p. 15, where excretion via
the urine is discussed.

5–6 smoky vapors: Probably end-products of metabolism. "Vapors" are also
mentioned by Galen; see introduction, p. 15 and medical contents, p. 20.

9–10 two drams per ounce: The prescription of drugs in precise weights and
measures is much more common in medieval medical literature than in
ancient medicine.

11 dilation of the spirit: See our note to 133r, 8*.

12 When the physicians speak: The use of oxtongue must have been widely
known and accepted in the medical practice of the time.

---

* When this volume was ready for press we were presented with the learned M.Sc. thesis of N.
Shlamovitz (See bibliography). The effects, in animal experiments, show "phenomena similar
to those produced by tranquilizers", when injected but not when given per os. — The plant
used was *Anchusa strigosa* and it is possible that Maimonides and the previous authors refer
to one of the other species of *Anchusa*.

והשמחה ושתיית היין מרטב הגוף 1
רטיבות כבר זכר גלינוס זה
בספרו בהנהגת הבריאות'
ואמנם מי שחשב שהוא מחמם
כבר טעה שהיין מזון לא רפואה 5
והוא מזון טוב מאד והמזונות
הטובים אינם מחממין ולא מקררין
והרפואות הן שמחממות ומקררות משונה
ולא יתילד ממנו כי אם דם משובח
בטבע הדם הטבע שהוא חם 10
ולח · ואמנם מזיגתו בלי ספק
מולידה הרוחות ולפעמים עליה
רעש וכבר זכר זה אבן זהר
והוא היחיד שברורו ומגדולי

1 and the delight of the spirit. Drinking wine moistens the body with a good moisture; Galen has already mentioned this in his book on the regimen of health.

5   Whoever assumed that it heats, was mistaken, for wine is a nutrient, not a medicament. It is a very good nutrient, and the good nutriments neither heat nor cool; it is the medicaments that heat and cool. Indeed, it generates

10 praiseworthy blood, of the nature of the natural blood, which is hot and wet. As to mixing it, there is no doubt that this will generate flatus, and could possibly generate tremor. Nevertheless, Ibn Zuhr, who was unique in his age and one of the greatest sages,

5–8 a nutrient not a medicament: Drugs were regarded as substances which altered the four cardinal properties (cold, heat, and so on), while nutriments were neutral in this regard. Wine is here considered as a good nutriment and one that "generates praiseworthy blood."

11 As to mixing it: When wine was mixed with water of oxtongue, it was considered to be a drug which could produce undesirable side effects (flatulence and tremor) when drunk immediately after it was mixed.

13 Ibn Zuhr: The advice is given on the authority of Abū Marwān ibn Zuhr (? 1091 to ? 1161), whom Maimonides also quotes in his *Aphorisms* (particula 22).

הרופאים שהמזון ישנה זה כשימזג אותו

לשעתו וישתהו אבל אם הונח שהם עשרה

שעות או יותר ואז ישתה יהיה אז טוב

מאד שהייעת תתחזק על הקימית

ותחולנגה ותיפה המזג וממה שמיע

בן העבד הוא שהראו להעשות מלשון

השור הוא קליפות שרשין לא עלהו כמן ‏עלי

שעושין אנשי ארץ ישר ואנשי מצריס

כך ראינו כל הזקינים המשובחים

עושים בספרד וכל הערב אינם מזכירי

כי אם קליפת שרשין לא עלין וזה צימח

ראוי לאדועט שלא יעזבנו מפני שישלו

סגולה בהרחיב הנפש ומחיית הלחה ‏המרה

ה שחורה והסרת פעולתה וממה

שנסה ה עבד אותן ונתאמת אימות

אימות אין ספק בן שהיין הדק ימצ

1

5

10

15

2: שהם] Should read שתים.   7: עלהו] In the margin עליו (in MS. Berlin העלים).   8: וישר]
Abbreviation of ישראל.   10: מזכירי] Abbreviation of מזכירים.   12: יעזבנו.   13: הלחה]
In the margin המרה.   16: אימות] word repeated by mistake.   כשיומזג.

1   has already mentioned that the mixture does this if it is mixed and drunk
at once, but if mixed and left for twelve hours or more and then drunk, it
5   is very good, since the vinous part surmounts the watery and alters it, and
the temperament improves.

This Servant suggests that what ought to be used of the oxtongue is the
bark of its roots, not its leaves as the people of Syria and the people of
10   Egypt do; thus we have seen all the outstanding Elders do in the land of
Andalusia. And all the Arabs prescribe the bark of its roots, not its leaves.
Our Master should not neglect this herb, because it has the virtue of dilating
the spirit, effacing the black humor and eradicating its traces.
15   This Servant has tried and verified as true, without any doubt, that light
wine, if mixed

1–5   Thus a tincture is made of the drug: an alcoholic solution usually diluted
with water. The assumption is also expressed that on prolonged contact
with wine, the drug is altered (possibly the side effects are thereby mitigated).
Again in the *Aphorisms* (particula 21), Maimonides refers to vinous and
watery parts in a beverage, as here (line 4).

8   Syria: The Hebrew text reads "the land of Israel." The Latin manuscripts
seem to refer to the town of Acre, although the readings are by no means
clear. Most suggestive of this is the word *accho* in the Vienna manuscript.
This spelling for Acre in Greek characters is to be found in: Hadrianus
Relandus. 1714, p. 534.

במעט מי ורד שא שיעור העשור הוא

מרחיב הנפש ולא ישבר ולא יזיק למוח

הראש ויחזק הא׳ צו ומכא ומוסיף בכל

השבחיס המיוחסיס ליין לפ׳ יועץ

העבר שיושס באוקיה הכנענית עשר

דרהם מי הורד ועשרים דרהם מי

לשון שור ניונח עשר שעת או קרוב ·

להנואז יוקח · ואמנם לקיחתן גם

כן כשעת השינה עצה טובה מפני

פעס רבים שישקע בשינה ויסיר

המחשבה ומיתה העיכול נדחה

היתרונות · פרק / ואמנם מב

הסכמת הרופאיס על היות המזג

כבר נטה אל החמימות וראוי שיקח

מה שיקרר ומרטב זה מאמר אמת

1: **במעט**. 2: **ישבר**] Should read **ישכר**. 4: **לפי**] Abbreviation of **לפיכך**. 5: **עשׂר**] Abbreviation of **עשרה**.

with a little rose water, about a tenth, will dilate the spirit, will not inebriate, will not harm the brain, will strengthen the stomach and augment
5 all the virtues associated with wine. Therefore, this Servant recommends steeping twenty drams of oxtongue in one Syrian ounce of wine and ten drams of rose water. It should be left for about ten hours, and then it should be taken. As to taking it also at bedtime, this is an excellent idea for
10 various reasons; sleep deepens, anxiety departs, the digestion improves and the superfluities are repelled.

The consensus of the physicians that when the temperament tends to-   Chapter 3
15 ward the hot one should take something to cool and moisten, is correct,

2 will not harm the brain: Because the Sultan as a Muslim may not be acquainted with the effects of drinking wine, the author reassures him that no harm will ensue when the wine is taken in the prescribed manner.

4 virtue: The Jerusalem Hebrew manuscript translates the word as "praise" (*shevaḥ*) and the Berlin manuscript as "merits" (*ma'alot*).

8–12 Various effects on bodily functions are attributed to oxtongue. The psychopharmacological effect is mentioned by Galen; see our comment on 133*r*, 8.

12 Here begins Chapter 3, chiefly on the "temperaments."

13 The consensus of the physicians: The humoral theory, with its four qualities and properties, was generally accepted by the physicians of the period and used to explain all bodily and psychic conditions.

אבל הוא כלי ראוי שיפורט ולהזכיר ——

ההנהגה   ואמנם מי שיען מהם

בשתיית מי העולשין ומשקה העול

ומשרת התמר הנדי ואגוז וזיזב

יראה לעבד צדה חטא גדול שאן

ההנהגה הסוחלנת עם היות

הלחה הלבנה יש לה התגברות ממזג

העיקרי אינה ראויה בשום פנס

וכלבד באפרושן והדזב שזה מרפה

האצטומכא ומזיק לה מאד ומקרר

העכולים   וכשתתרעב האצטומכא

ותתרפה יפסדו העכולים השלשה

ואינה ראויה זו ההנהגה לא למי

1: שיפורט.   3: הצודל [Should read הצנדל.   4: וזיב.   12: ותתרפה.

60

1 but their statement was too brief; it ought to be detailed and the regimen mentioned.

Whoever advocated drinking water of endive in sandalwood syrup, and
5 the infusion of tamarind, prunes, and jujubes, appears to this Servant to be in grave error, because, although phlegm is dominant in the original temperament, this general regimen is not at all suitable, especially the
10 prunes and the jujubes. It will debilitate the stomach, harm it greatly, and curtail the digestion, and whenever the stomach is moistened and debilitated, the three digestions are corrupted. The like of this regimen is not suitable except for one

1–2 it ought to be detailed and the regimen mentioned: Here the practical medical approach of the author is substantiated by an analysis of the supposedly "hot temperament" and by an enumeration of the merits and disadvantages of the diet recommended for this "temperament."

9 Plums and certain other fruits are rejected as exerting a bad effect on the stomach and bowels, although they would be acceptable for cooling the temperament.

10–11 curtail the digestion: The rejection of this prescription is probably based on its predominantly purgative effect, which precludes proper absorption of the ingested food.

12 the three digestions: The assimilation of food in the stomach, in the liver, and in the organs of the body.

שׁברה עליו המרה האדומה

ולא זכר שום דבר שמורה על

התגברות המרה האדומה

בשום פעם אלא הנלקח מכל

הראיין הנזכרות הוא התילדות

אדים שחורים שנהוין ממרה

שחורה מתילדת משריסתלחת

לחה לבנה שבאה במשמרות׳

פרק   ואמנם מי שיעץ בשתיית

משרת הראונד במי

העולשין יום אחד ועוד ב׳ ימים

אם כון כזה לרפות המעים הוא

נכון׳ וכבר זכר העבר שלשול

אדים שחורים 6:   שגברה 1:

1 who is dominated by yellow bile. Yet nothing is mentioned that indicates dominance of yellow bile at all, while the implication of the whole of the
5 indications mentioned is the generation of black vapors caused by the black bile arising from the combustion of phlegm that recurs periodically.
10 As to him who suggested drinking an infusion of rhubarb in water of   Chapter 4 endive one day and then abstaining for two, if he intended by that to soften the stools, then he is correct; this Servant has already mentioned the method of softening the stools

1 yellow bile: In the Hebrew text, the term is translated as red bile. In this condition laxatives were regarded as useful, and they are still prescribed in the management of biliary conditions.

7–8 combustion of phlegm: See 137*r* and 143*r*, 4, "inflammation [or combustion] of phlegm." The meaning of the term phlegm has been defined by Galen as follows: "When we look for the origin of the Greek word *phlegm*, it becomes evident that it stems from inflammation or combustion, because this temperament, which arises from the bile, is formed in this manner." This passage, taken from the treatise *On Medical Nomenclature*, a work which survives only in Arabic translation, bears some resemblance to our text. Galen also derives the term *phlegmonē*, a hot swelling, in a similar manner. See M. Meyerhof, 1928, p. 15.

בראונד בפרק הג ממאמרו שכבר 1
באככית אדוננו: פרק
ואמנם מי שיעץ בריחיצה בכל ג
מהימים והטיול בכליום והמשיחה
בשמן הבנפסג וכל זה נכון 5
וידבר העצב בתילוק ושיעור
פרק   ואמנם מי שיעץ בהנחת
המעליות המתענד לות
על הכבד וכמוכן מי שיעץ
באכילת המלפפון והחזרת 10
והקישואיס והרגלה והאספרגך
והקטף כל אן חטא גמור וזו
הנהגה ראויה לבעלי החממיות

1 with rhubarb, in the third chapter of his treatise that has already been presented in the court of our Master.

5   The suggestions for bathing every three days, exercising each day and anointing with oil of violets, are all correct; this Servant will speak about this clearly and adequately.   Chapter 5

He who advocated placing cloths with sandalwood upon the liver, and he   Chapter 6
10 also who advised eating cucumber, lettuce, snake cucumber, purslane, spinach and orach, are absolutely wrong, for this is a regimen that suits those who harbor the intensely inflaming

1 in the third chapter of his treatise: That is, the *Regimen*. This is a further indication that our treatise was written later than the *Regimen* and was addressed to the same Sultan.

3–6 The chapter on bathing is very brief. This is probably because the subject belonged to the accepted practice of hygiene at the time of Maimonides, and he had nothing to add to the opinions expressed by the court physicians.

4 Exercising and anointing were closely connected with the practice of warm bathing.

6 will speak: Probably the author is referring to his twenty-first chapter, in which he briefly mentions bathing, exercising, sleep, diet, and the regimen in winter and summer.

8 cloths with sandalwood: That is, poultices to be placed on the liver. These were rejected by the author because of incompatibility with the patient's constitution. Various medical indications for the use of sandalwood are cited by Lane, I, Pt. IV, p. 1732.

1   השורפות והחזקות בהתהלכות

כשיארע לחמי המזג בק״ץ

ויותר מזה חטא מי שיעץ ~

בשתיתה החלב החלוב עיין ~

5   כעניין השלשול ושכח מהירות

פסידותן לאי זו לחה שימצא

ולא זכר כמו מר עכת החלי ~

והיא הלחה השרופה׃   פרק

ומי שיעץ בעשיית

10   הסכנגבן אחר המזון בשעה

הוא נכון והנהגה טובה מיפה

העיכולים ׃ ואמנם תוספתו ~

למשקה שחיתברכאריס אחד

[אחד   .ברבאריס or ברבריס   13:   [ברכאריס Should read ברבריס   .בהתהלכות [בההתהלכות :1

Spelling mistake; should be אחר.

1 burning fevers, should these occur in those of hot temperament in the
summer. More grave is the error of the one who advises drinking fresh
5 milk, because he has caught a glimpse of its moistening virtue, over-
looked its quick transformation into any humor whatever, and failed to
consider the essence of the cause of this disease, which is the inflamed
phlegm.
10 He who advised the use of oxymel of quince an hour after the meal, is   Chapter 7
correct; it is a good regimen to improve the digestion. But adding it to a
drink of barberry extract

2 in the summer: Special dietary rules for the various seasons of the year are
very common in ancient and medieval literature; for example, in the *Regimen
of Salerno*. See also the long poem by Abraham Ibn Ezra, "The Regimen of
Health," (1894, I: 180–186).

4 fresh milk: Is not recommended because of its possible "transformation"
(line 6). However, in the *Regimen*, Chapter I (in Bar-Sela's translation, p. 19),
Maimonides writes: "Freshly drawn milk is a good nutrient for those in
whom it does not sour in the stomach."

6 any humor whatever: The Paris Hebrew manuscript here adds "in the
stomach."

4–8 On milk and its medical properties see: Dioscorides, II, Chapters 75–78. The
same subject is discussed at greater length by Maimonides in his *Aphorisms*,
Section 20 (in the Muntner Hebrew edition, pp. 232–233).

8 inflamed phlegm: See note to 136*r*, lines 6–8. Possibly Maimonides refers to
milk fresh from the cow, hence to unboiled milk that is thus likely to be
infected and to give rise to "inflamed phlegm."

10 Oxymel in various combinations with currants or roses is mentioned later in
the treatise as being beneficial in urinary disorders. Its mode of action is
described in the *Regimen*, Chapter 3: "for the vinegar in the oxymel cuts
the phlegm and opposes putrefaction of the humors."

אחר המאכל זו הנהגה זרה יוצאה

מההיקשים הרפואותיים

ומהמורגל רעו לומ לקיחת שחיתת

הברברים זה המאכל כאיעומלא

עד שאפי היה האיעזומלא פניה

אז יפתח לשחיטה כזה החלי.

פרק ואמנם מי שיעץ במשאך

המשמח שלאק הת

התלמיד אז זולתו וכמו כן מי שיעץ

במשקה המשמה כתומאן ותפוחים

ומי לשון השור וזרע הדס וזרע

תרנואן כל זה נכון ואמנם

הוספתו לזה בזרקטונא אינו

1
5
10

1: אחר] Repeated by mistake.   3: רצו לומ] Abbreviation of רצוני לומר.   5: שאפי] Abbreviation of שאפילו.   7: במשקה.   8: שלאק] Should read של אבן.   [הת'] Canceled by the scribe.
10: במשקה המשמח] Canceled by the scribe, but the word המשקה must be retained according
to the Arabic text.   12: תרנואן] Should read תרנגאן.   13: אינו] After this, the word רואה
(يراة) should be added.

68

1 after the meal is an uncommon regimen not in accord with medical regu-
   lations and custom, that is, taking barberry extract while the food is in the
5 stomach. Even when the stomach is empty, the extract should not be introduced in this disease.

   Whoever suggested drinking the exhilarating drink of Ibn al-Talmid or   Chapter 8
10 someone else, and likewise he who advised syrup of sorrel, apples, water of
   oxtongue, seeds of basil and seeds of the balm gentle, are all correct. But
   this Servant does not see the point of adding the seeds of fleabane

1–6 Here the difference is noted between the physiological reaction of the stomach
     when it contains food and when it is empty.

4   On the medicinal properties of barberry, see *Regimen*, Chapter 3.

7–8 The exhilarating drink: Contains substances thought to exert psychophar-
     macological effects.

9   On the Christian Arab physician Ibn al-Tilmīdh who lived in Baghdad at
     the end of the 11th century, see *Encyclopedia of Islam*, 1969, III: 956.

13   fleabane: *Plantago psyllium* L. In the excavations in the Judean Desert caves,
     fleabane seeds from the time of Bar-Kokba, second century A.D., were
     found among other medicinal drugs in the possession of the besieged popu-
     lation (Dr. Zaitschek), showing the importance which was attributed to
     psyllium in those times.
        The toxicity of fleabane is mentioned in a pseudo-Dioscoridic treatise,
     translated by J. Berendes, 1907, where it is included among the deadly poisons,
     p. 407, Cap. 145. See also note to 138*r*, line 1.
        The drug was mentioned in the thirteenth-century Hebrew work *Ha-
     mebakesh* by Falaqera, 1778, (p. 16 A), under the same name, *basar katuna*,
     as in our manuscript. This author notes that under some circumstances it
     can be highly toxic.

69

אותן ה עבד שאנו אינו רואה כהקרר 1
רב כוה החלי וזה המזג פרק
ואמנם מי שיעץ כלקיחת מי השעורי
כבשכש וזרע יקטיץ הוא פלא עז מה
שזכר מהשוית השינה והיה אצלו 5
רתיכות הרכה מקצרה ע''
שסמכה כזרע היקטין ויותר
פלא מזה מי שראה כלקיחת ~/
האפרועם אחר מי השעורין אינו
מחשב שיש אצל או הרופאים 10
אכר מאכרי הגוף יותר פחות
מהא צטומכא ושאין ראוי ~/
לפנות לאצטומכא נתרפנה ~

3: השעורי] Abbreviation of השעורים.   4: יקטץ] Should read יקטין.   עז] Should read עם.
13: נתרפנה] Should read נתרפתה.

1   because I cannot visualize a rigorous regimen in this disease and this temperament.

The suggestion by one physician to take barley water with poppy and
5   seeds of round pumpkin is surprising, even though he has mentioned the
moderation of sleep, and maintains that the moistening effect of barley
water is insufficient, so that he has supplemented it with the seeds of round
pumpkin. More surprising than this is the suggestion to take prunes follow-
10   ing the barley water. I do not suppose that for these physicians there is
any member of the body more lowly than the stomach, or that they take
into consideration whether the stomach is debilitated

1   a rigorous regimen: Our Arabic consultant notes that the author rejects the
advice of the other physicians to use *psyllium* because it possesses "cooling"
properties. In the Arabic manuscripts, other than that published by Kroner,
the word *tabrīd* ("cooling") appears; this also conforms with the Hebrew
version, *hekrer* (*kirūr*). Galen, in his *De simplicium medicamentorum tempe-*
ramentis, Book VIII, Chapter 23, 2 (K. XII: 158), says that *psyllium* "cools
and dries" in the second degree. Excessive cooling was not regarded by the
author as an appropriate measure "in this disease and this temperament,"
as explicitly noted in 143r, 3.

The term excessive cooling is also used to denote intoxication. As Ibn al-
Bayṭār puts it: "When psyllium is taken in excess, the whole body becomes
cool; loss of consciousness and fainting will come" (Sontheimer edition, I:
132–133). He quotes this from a work which he attributes to Dioscorides,
although it is in fact apocryphal. See our note to 137v, line 13.

3   barley water: Often used as a vehicle for medication. As late as 1556, Amatus
Lusitanus used barley water in this manner for the treatment of a gastric
condition, which I have interpreted as a probable peptic ulcer (Leibowitz,
1953).

4   poppy: It is rejected not only because of its toxicity, but also as unnecessary,
because the patient's sleep was regular (Arabic: balanced), a fact documented
on 143v, 9: "It is wholly a blessing that sleep is regular."

9–10   I do not suppose: The importance of a thorough knowledge of gastric disease
is stressed by the author. See our introduction, p. 16).

או לא נתרפתה אירעה בה מכה או

לא אירעה אן שמא הם מודיס

בשיאות האיצטומכא וכלל

תעלתה ושראני להשגיח בה תמיד

ולפי הפרידו כל משובחי הרופאיס

לה מאמרות לא שזו ההנהגה אעלם בגלותה

מחזקת האיצטומכא ומיבשת

ומחתכת התרבקות הלחה הלבנה

שאינה פוסקת מלהתקבץ בה

תמיד והיא כיתה ומדיקקת

עביותה והיא ההנהגה אקדיס

זכרונה אצלם והיא מי השעריס

כזרע היקטן והכשכאש ויפעיר

אחריה כאפרועם ולא הוציא דבה

הّעَבَّ

1

5

10

5: ‏ולפי] After this word, זה should be added.   13: ‏היקטן] Should read היקטין.

72

1   or not, and whether there is moistness in it or not. Perhaps they do acknowledge the nobility of the stomach and its general usefulness, and that care
5   should always be given to it, for which reason the best physicians have
devoted treatises to it. Nevertheless, according to the former, the regimen
previously mentioned by them, that is, barley water with seeds of round
pumpkin, poppy, and the subsequent taking of prunes, will strengthen the
stomach, improve its digestion, dry its moistness, cut the viscidity of the
10 phlegm which evidently never ceases accumulating in it, and thin its thickness.

1   moistness: Our Hebrew version gives the term *makkah*, which would denote
an organic lesion, in this case of the stomach. This accords with the Paris
manuscript (Arabic in Hebrew letters), but not with the two manuscripts
written in Arabic characters, where the Arabic term can only denote "moistness." The term used in the Paris text, as well as in the Hebrew version, may
allude to peptic ulcer, a diagnosis which is quite unusual for the state of
medical knowledge during the twelfth and thirteenth centuries. See the
medical thesis of our student Avishai Teicher (1970).

7   dry its moistness: Barley is referred to by Hippocrates very often, *inter alia*
in the *Regimen*, Book 2, xl, where barley cakes are also mentioned.

8   cut the viscidity of the phlegm: This refers to the mucus which tends to
accumulate in the stomach in some forms of gastritis.

13 The mixing of barley water with a strong ingredient such as poppy, is rejected
by the author.

Note: In the English translation, lines 6–14, the regimen and its effects have been transposed,
unlike the original Arabic, the Hebrew version. and the Latin and Kroner's translations.

העבד בזה הפרק מה שראוי לפסמו   1
כיֵים להשמר מאד ואל ישגיח ~
למאמר אומרן כלל ·   פרק

ויֵמנם לקיחת התפוחים והחבושם
ומעיצת גרעיני הרימונים אחר   5
המאכל לא מצווה בהם כחוק כב
אדם כולם כהנהגת הבריאות·
ואין בזה תוספת ותלית בזה החלי
לא מה שזכר מלקיחת כמברחמ
אחר המאכל זה שחוק בֵאמתות   10
שאומר זה אמרן מפני היות קברחמ
מעכבה האדים ומונעת אותם
מלעלות וזה אמת אבל היא ~
ראוייה שתיקח במסמֵין כשתֵיחֵת

1   This Servant censures in this section what ought to be censured only in
order to warn strongly, not because he is inclined to make such statements
in general.

5   Taking apple and quince, and sucking pomegranate seeds after the meal   Chapter 10
are recommended for everyone as part of the regimen of health.
There is nothing superfluous in it in relation to this disease, except what

10 was mentioned regarding taking coriander following the meal. This is
truly laughable. This was proposed because coriander thickens the vapors
and prevents their ascent, which is right, but it ought to be taken in medicaments like medicinal powders

11   coriander thickens the vapors and prevents their ascent: About coriander,
see Galen, *De simplicium medicamentorum temperamentis ac facultatibus*, Book
VII, Chapter 10, 43 (K. XII: 36 ff.) and Dioscorides, III, 64 [71]. Ibn al-
Baytār (Sontheimer, II: 373–377) provides a long exposition on the medicinal
properties of coriander compiled from ancient and medieval authors. Although "vapors" are not mentioned, an ascent (Hebrew MS. Berlin adds:
to the brain) is implied by the quotation from Dioscorides to the effect that
"when taken in excess it disturbs the mind."

14   it ought to be taken in medicaments: The author does not oppose the use of
coriander, but stresses that it should be taken "in medicaments . . . or cooked
with the food." This remark accords with his general rule set down in 135v:
"It ought to be detailed and the regimen mentioned."

ודימיהן או תבושל עם המזונות
אכל לקיחת הכסברתא לבדה אחר
המאכל אם לא יביא קיא הוא מביא
רצון הקיא בלי ספק ומפסיד
המאכל   ואמנם לקיחת זרע
הרגלה בסוכר בקצת העתים
לא עם המאכל זה טוב ואפי׳
עתערב עם המאכל גם כן לא
הזיק זה בקרירותו והחזקתו
ללב   פרק   וזכר אדוננו שיעמן
הרופאיס בלקיחת המשמש
והכמתרא והחבנשיס אחר
המאכל והענבים והאצטחיס
והתאנים והר כונעם לפנו ולא ידע

7: ‏ואפי׳] Abbreviation of ‏ואפילו.   12: ‏והכמתרא] Mistake corrected by a later hand.
14: ‏והתאנים] Missing in the Arabic text and in MS. Berlin.

76

1   and the like, or cooked with the food. As to taking coriander alone after
the meal, if it does not cause vomiting it will undoubtedly cause nausea
5   and corrupt the meal. Occasionally taking purslane seeds in sugar apart
from the meal is good. Taken with the meal these also cause no harm
10 because they cool and strengthen the heart.

Our Master has mentioned that the physicians advised taking apricots,   Chapter 11
pears, and quinces after the meal, and grapes, melons, and pomegranates
before it. This Servant does not understand

2–4   As to taking coriander: In such a way the quantity of coriander is small and
does no harm, while taken alone it might produce toxic effects.

9–10   Purslane: It is thought to strengthen the heart because of its cooling properties. Throughout the treatise, cardiac dyscrasia is considered to be due
to the overheating of this organ.

העבד ענין העצ֞ אם היתה 1

הכונה שהדריכה התאוה והמנהג

ללקיחת מעט מהפירנה ראוי שיקח

קודם ⬦ המאכל מה שמרפה

המעים ויאחר מהפירות אחר 5

המאכל מה שיש בו אימוץ

ככמהתא והכבושיס והתפוחים

וזה נכון ואם הם יעצנ שלקיחת

הפירות מועלים לזה תחל והחוץ

שהפירות הרטובים בלם רעם 10

לכל הבריאים ולחולים ⬦ כשיוקחו

על דרך המזון ובלבד האבחים

והכמש ההפסדות שלהם לאי ח

לחה רעה שתהיה בגוף וכמוק

1: וו] Added by the same hand, which also corrected העצם to העצה.   3: מהפירנה] Should read מהפירות.   7: ככמהתא] Should read ככמתרא; corrected in the manuscript by a later hand.

1   the intent of this advice. If there was need to induce appetite, or a habit of taking fruits, the intent is correct, and thus one should take before the

5   meal whatever soften the stools and after the meal those fruits in which there is astringence, like pear, quince, and apple. But if they advised that

10   taking these fruits is beneficial in this disease, this is an error, for all the fresh fruits are bad for everyone, healthy or sick, if taken as nutrients, and especially the melon and the apricot, because of the rapidity of their change into whatever evil humor there is in the body.

8   The author admits that the advice given by the other physicians is correct in principle, but it does not suit the special condition of the patient.

10–14   The author's rejection of "soft fruit" (in Hebrew: "moist fruit") is more clearly explained in his *Regimen*, Chapter 1 (Bar-Sela's translation, p. 20); "The superfluities of their juices will remain in the veins mixed with the blood, and will boil. This is a major factor in the generation of putrid fevers." The author returns to this problem in his *Mishneh Torah*, Book of knowledge, (*Hilkot de'ot*), Chapter 4, § 11. (See English translation by Hyamson, 1937, p.51a). In this work, which Maimonides wrote in Hebrew, he refers to "moist fruits," the same words used in our Hebrew text, although Hyamson translates the term as "fresh fruits." That the ingestion of fruit may induce fever is also mentioned on 140*v*, 3.

     Similar opinions regarding soft fruits were also voiced by Abū Marwān Ibn Zuhr, whom Maimonides held in high esteem. See Ibn Zuhr's *De nutrimentis*, Hebrew translation, MS. Munich 220[1], p. 14; Ibn Zuhr based his opposition on Galen's authority (see our medical contents on p. 22). The opposition is understandable because of the rapid spoilage of soft fruit in a hot country such as Egypt.

האפרסקין רע מאד והן חומר חמימות

הרעים הגדולים וכבר זכר גאלינס

שהוא מעת שהפסיק מאכל לא נתחמס

עד סוף ימין והאריך בספור שלו

לפי ראוי שירחיק אדונגו הפירות

הלחים כל יכלתו :   פרק

ומי שיעץ להרחיק בשר

הצייר והבשר המליח והעככיות ועל

כה שמחמס כבר קישיר וכל זה

מוסיף במה שקבל ממגו אדונגו

מהמקריס וכמו כן מי שיעץ טיול

בכליוס הפיק רצון מאד וכמו כן

מי שהזהיר מההליכה לארכות

החמות מחוללות האדים אכות

בעבתן ואמנם מי שחשב הואר צות

2: גאלינוס.   3: מאכול] The ו added by a later hand.   3: אותם] Added in the manuscript by a later hand.   5: לפי] Abbreviation of לפיכך.   6: בכל] ב added in the manuscript by a later hand.   8: הצייר] Should read הצייד.

80

1   The peach is also very evil and it is the substance of the evil malignant
    fevers. Galen has already mentioned that since he stopped eating all fresh
    fruits, he had not had a fever to the end of his life; he dilated on this story
5   of his as an admonition to everyone, as expressed in his treatise. Therefore,
    it behooves our Master to avoid fresh fruits all he can.

    He spoke the truth who advocated avoidance of game meat, cured meat,   Chapter 12
10 eggplant, and everything that heats, for all these increase those accidents
    of which our Master has complained. The one who suggested exercising
    every day gave most appropriate advice. Likewise, he who forbade travel
15 to the hot regions gave good advice in his suggestion. He who assumed that
    hot regions

2–4   Galen has already mentioned: According to Hebrew MS. Berlin, it was
      mentioned "in his treatise on hygiene" (that is, in *De sanitate tuenda*), an
      addition not present in the Arabic texts nor in our manuscript. In the
      Regimen, the wording is: "until his father forbade him to eat any fruit at all,
      and he was saved from the fever that year." In *De sanitate tuenda* Galen indeed
      notes that he overcame his childhood predisposition to sickness by adherence to
      the rules of hygiene (K. VI, 309). However, the parts of the story concerning
      his father and the fruit only occur in *De probis pravisque alimentorum succis*,
      Chapter 1 (K. VI: 755 ff.).

8   cured meat (Arabic—*alqadīd*): Salted meat, dried in the sun after it is cut
      into long strips.
      eggplant: According to Galen, this is "hot in the third degree" and was
      therefore not regarded as suitable for the patient.

החמות מחוללות האדים הם שֻׁעָלִים   1
לשעת הגוף זה כשיהיו קרים לחים ~
אבל זו העליה שהיא מדם עבה עכור
אותן הארצות מוסיפות בעוביהדם
ואורפות אותן ומוסיפות אדין ·   5
וכשיתבונן בריאות בעז' הא' ילך
אדונען לאיזה מקום שירצה במקום
שישלים כל רצונו בשע עולמות:
פרק   ואינן רואה העב
כהחרקה באזורד ולא   10
כאבן הארמיני האזורד מפני
והאבן הארמיע מפע היותן מוס כל
העין וכבר נסתפקו בן ורובם
שאינן זה שקוראין אותן כזה השם
וכמו כן יישיר העבד עצת מי שהזהיר   15

1: שֻׁעָלִים] Should read שעולים .5: אידיו. 6: וכשיתבונן] Should read וכשיתכונן. [בעז
הארמיני .11: בלאזורד] Corrected by a later hand to באזורד .10: בעזרת Abbreviation of
After this, a mark has been added by a later hand. האזורד] Corrected by the same later
hand to הלאזורד .13: נסתפקו בו] After this, the words טובי הרופאים should be added,
according to the Arabic text.

82

1 melt the vapors is correct only with respect to those vapors that ascend
to the surface of the body if they are cool and moist. As to those that arise
from thick turbid blood, such regions would only augment the thickness
5 of the blood and its inflammation, and increase its vapors. When health
is reestablished, as God wills, our Master may travel wherever he wishes,
until God grants his hopes in the two worlds.

10 This Servant does not approve of emesis with lapis lazuli or with the Chapter 13
Armenian stone; with the lapis lazuli because of its vehemence, and with
the Armenian stone because it is of obscure substance. The accomplished
among the physicians, most of them, have already had doubts regarding
15 the latter, whether it is what is designated by this name. This Servant
approves the view of whomever it was who admonished

 1 hot regions: About hemoconcentration, see our introduction, pp. 14–15.

1–4 vapors that ascend to the surface of the body if they are cool and moist:
See *Galeni adversus Lycum libellus*, II, (K. XVIII A: 205–206), where Galen
seems to differentiate between insensible and sensible perspiration. See also
B. Castellus, *Dictionary*, (1746), *s.v.* Diapnoe, p. 258.

 5 inflammation: In the Arabic manuscripts, Paris and Huntington, "And burn
it" (the blood) and thereby increase its vapors.

6–8 When health is reestablished: Restrictions of a medical nature are to be
abolished if the patient recovers.

 10 lapis lazuli: According to Ibn al-Baytār, on Galen's authority, it possesses
astringent qualities.

12–13 obscure substance: In both Arabic and Hebrew, "obscure to the eye."

מעשית המשלשלים החזקים והקיצור 1

על הראוונד או מי הגבינה או ~

הסנא המכי ודומיהן כל זה נכון

ואינן רואה העובד כמשרת ~

האפרסקין ולא כמי האבטחים 5

להזיקתם כאצטומכא ואין במה

שק כל מה מקרים לא התלהבות

ולא צמאון ואינן רואה גם כן ~

בהרבאה מהעלוקר מפע

שמענה הדס ומרפא ~ 10

האצטומכא ואינן ראוי זה כי

אם לבעלי החמימיות החדות

המתלהבות כמו שזכר העבד

ואינן רואה העובד גם כן בעשית

7: התלהבות.   10: ומרפא [ומרפה] Corrected in the manuscript to ומרפה.

1 against the employment of strong purgatives, and advised restriction to rhubarb or whey or senna of Mecca and the like; all of this is correct.

5 This Servant does not approve the infusion of peaches or melon juice, because of their harm to the stomach; there is not, in those accidents complained of, either burning or thirst. He also does not approve the

10 excessive use of water lily, because it thickens the blood and debilitates the stomach; this suits only those who have acute inflammatory fevers, as this Servant has mentioned. Moreover this Servant sees no point in the use of

2–3 purgatives: Although rhubarb and senna have a long reputation as laxatives, whey is uncommon for this purpose in older sources but is approved in household medicine.

6 harm to the stomach: The cautious physician considers possible side effects.

9 water lily: The Hebrew translator uses the Arabic term *nīlūfar*. This substance was rejected by the author, because "it thickens the blood" (see our introduction, p. 14). The possibility of harmful side effects of the treatment is often considered in this treatise. Water lily is mentioned together with ox-tongue on 143*r*, 7. If their effects on the body are also thought to be similar, then a diuretic property such as ascribed to oxtongue (133*v*, 4–7) might be presupposed for water lily as well.

בישול האפיתמון מפני הכאבתו 1
והיבשתו ואם הושרה האפיתמון
בק דרהס ממי הגביה ולוקח
זה פעמים שלא בזמן ניסן ופעם
ביומי תשרי או פעמים יהיה עוב 5
ויהיה בין כל פעם שׁן יוס ובוללין
האפיתמון בשמן שקדים ועורין
אותו במשלית קלה ואחר כן שורין
אותו לילה בני הגבה · פרק
וזכר אדועו שכבר הקיז 10
(הגד פעסו ועו הדס עבה כמו
העחול ועעו הרופאיס מפע זה
בהקזה · אמנס לפי מה שיראה
בעת זולת עת מההתמלאות יתחייב

4: פעמים] After this, the word או should be added. שלא] Corrected in the manuscript by a later hand to שלש. 5: ביומי. 9: הגבנה] Should read הגבינה.

1 cooked dodder of thyme because of its distressing and drying action. If the dodder of thyme is infused in a hundred drams of whey, and taken
5 twice or three times in the springtime and once or twice in the autumn, it is good, but there should be fifteen days between one time and the other. The dodder of thyme should be crumbled in almond oil, wrapped in fine cloth, and then steeped overnight in the whey.
10 Our Master mentioned that a vessel had once been opened, and there came out blood as thick as spleen, whereupon the physicians counseled on this account, further bloodletting. In so far as plethora appears at one time or another,

Chapter 14

1–9 The detailed exposition reveals the cautious attitude of the author toward the administration of potentially harmful drugs.

2 drying action: See the commentary to Paulus Aegineta by Francis Adams, III: 111.

10–13 blood as thick as spleen: This description and the proposed treatment by bloodletting (142*v*, 1) suggest that the author was dealing with the condition later known as polycythemia.

14 plethora: In classical Latin, *pletura* ("fullness"), for which bloodletting is advised.

בלי ספק שיקיז ויועיא מהורס לפיהן 1
ומה שראוי לכוין אותן תמיד הוא ~
סימון הדס והשיות מזגה כבד עד
שיוליד דס עוב וכבר באר העבד
כמאמרן הקורס היאך יהיה זה 5
במשקים שהרכיבם: פרק
ואמנם מי שיען כהיות
המזונים אפרסקיה ותמר הנדי ~
בבשר הגדייס זה נכון בזמן הקיץ
וראוי שלא יתעלם מהשמות האדרעיע 10
והמעטא והסנבל כאן התבשילין
ורומיהן עד שלא וזיקן לא צעומכא
וכמו כן ליקיחת מבושלקים המקדריס
כמו שיעשו בזמן הקיא שזה מיטה

10: הדארציני [האדרציני Should read.   14: הקיא [הקיץ Should read.

1 bloodletting is undoubtedly required, and the blood should be withdrawn proportionally. What should be aimed at always is clarification of the blood and rectification of the temperament of the liver so that good blood
5 is generated; the Servant has already explained in his previous treatise how this can be brought about through the syrups that he has compounded.

He who suggested that the nourishment should consist of peach and   Chapter 15 tamarind with the meat of the kid is correct for the summertime. We should
10 not neglect steeping cinnamon, mastic, nard, and the like, in these dishes, in order not to harm the stomach. On the other hand, taking cooling concoctions as they have counseled, in the summertime, could be disastrous

3   clarification of the blood: Probably hemodilution following venesection.

4   rectification of the temperament of the liver: According to Galenic physiology, the generation of "good blood" was dependent on the proper functioning of the liver (lines 3–4).

5   his previous treatise: The *Regimen*.

7   The next lines are devoted to diet. The fact that they follow immediately after the discussion of "plethora" and its supposed dependence on the "temperament of the liver" suggests some notion of the influence of nutrition on the composition of the blood.

12 not to harm the stomach: The author again stresses possible damage to this organ.

כתבתי אם לא ירבה מהן ולא ישכון ~ 1

כונה שעצת העבד השוית המזג לא

התוספת בקירור הואיל והעיקר ———

שרפות הלחה הלבנה · פרק

ואמנם מה שזכרו אדוננו 5

מרוב מה שעשה כלשון השור ———

והעלותו ולא נסתלק בזה עיקר ———

החלי הסכה במיעוט הועלתן רוב

התמרותן וכמו כן הסמנן החזקות

כשתותכמד עשיתן ירגיל אותן הטבע 10

ולא יפעל להן כלל ויהיו מזונות כבר

זכר זה גלינוס כל שכן אל הרפאות

החלושות הקרובות מן המזונות שהן

כשיוקחו שבוע נרדף ישלמון פעולות

הרפואיות ולא יראה להם אחר זה 15

2: כונה] Should read בכונה. 4: שרפאת] Should read שרפת. הלבנה] Following this, the text of Chapter 16, missing in this Hebrew manuscript, as copied from the Berlin Ms. or. quart. 836, 118v 3—6, reads: ואולם מי שייעץ בשתית השראב המשמח ובמרקחת יהיה בו יאקות. וזמראד וזהב וכסף הנה כל זה נכון ומועיל מאד לפי שהם סמים לביים יועילו בסגולה ר"ל בצורתם המינית אשר זה בכלל עצמותם לא באיכותם המופשט.

1   unless they are taken in moderation. They should not be taken deliberately, because this Servant's aim is the equilibration of the temperament, not an
4   increase in cooling, when the cause is inflammation of the phlegm.

The recommendation of exhilarating potions and the electuary in which   Chapter 16
there are jacinth, emerald, gold, and silver is correct and very beneficial, because these are cardiac medicaments which act through special properties, by which I mean their specific form which is the whole of their essence, and not through their particulars alone.

5   Our Master has mentioned his abundant use of oxtongue and water lily,   Chapter 17
despite which the cause of the disease has not disappeared. The reason for their limited effect is that they are continued too long. When the use of
10 extremely strong medicaments is continued, Nature becomes accustomed to them and she is no longer affected by them, and they turn into nourishment or the like of nourishment; Galen has already mentioned this. This is all the more so if these are weak medicaments, which are close to being nutriments. If these are taken continuously for a week, their medi-
15 cinal actions are abolished and not a trace of them appears thereafter.

---

3   increase in cooling: Refers to the concept that when the equilibrium of health has been restored, it should not be disturbed by excessive cooling measures.

4   inflammation of the phlegm: See our commentary to 136*r*, 6–8, referring to Galen's treatise on medical terminology, translated by Meyerhof, 1928.

After line 4, the short Chapter 16 is missing in the Jerusalem Hebrew manuscript, although it exists in the Berlin fragment.

to
Chap-
ter
16

The "exhilarating potions" mentioned in this passage are regarded as both psychotropic and cardiac medicaments; see our introduction. They act through "the whole of their essence" (in Hebrew: *segulah*) and were known as "sympathetic drugs," or "specifics," while their "properties" remained obscure. See our medical contents, p.24. The concept of specific property or form has been explained by Wellmann, 1928, and by Kraus, 1942.

On the medicinal use of gold see: Abraham Portaleone, 1584.

11–12 they turn into nourishment: See Galen, *De naturalibus facultatibus*, Book III, Chapter 8 (K. II: 161).

14–15 This refers to the fact that a diminished response to many drugs occurs when they are taken continuously.

לפי ראוי להעתק מרפואה לרפואה   1
ולהניח הרפואה האחת ימים ואז יחזור
לה   פרק   ואמנם מה שזכרו
אז ונגן מהרמעות

המשגל מההרגל זה טוב הפועל וכמה   5
גדולה תועלת זו ההמעשה ואמנם
המרחץ אין ראוי להנחו בשום פעמ׳
לא בעת המשמרת ולא בעת הפשרות
והיות השינה על המנהג זו טובה
שלימה וראיה ברורה שאן העשעם   10
השחורי׳ים לא הכעיסו למוח הראש
ולא שען מזגן ואולם מכאיבין הלב
בלבד׳ ואמנם מה שזכרו ארוגען
ממציאות הלשות אחר העיול

1   Therefore one ought to change from one medicine to another, or omit a medication for a few days and then return to it.

5   Our Master has mentioned a reduction in coitus from what was customary; this action is good, and what a great benefit comes from this reduction!

Chapter 18

The bath should never be neglected either during paroxysms of fever or during remissions.

10   It is wholly a blessing that sleep is regular, and a clear proof that these black vapors do not hurt the brain or alter its temperament, especially if the heart is afflicted.

As to what our Master has mentioned regarding the presence of weakness after exercise

1–2   In order to avoid drug habituation, the author advises changing medication or stopping the drug for a time.

3–6   For the general views of Maimonides on coitus, see his *Code* (*Mishneh Torah, Hilkot de'ot*, 4:19), in which he refers to the medically-beneficial aspects of sexual intercourse.

7–8   either during paroxysms of fever or during remissions: Bathing should not be discontinued, even during a febrile period. The Latin manuscript in the Friedenwald collection uses the contrasting expressions of "motus" and "quietis"; the Latin incunable uses "coytus—quietis."

10–12   black vapors: Black means melancholic. The author notes that the "vapors do not hurt the brain," because sleep is regular. However, according to our Hebrew version, they do particularly affect the heart. Cardiac symptoms such as "palpitation and throbbing" are mentioned later (145*r* and 148*r*).

11   vapors . . . brain: According to Galen, the thicker parts of the fuliginous residues are evacuated through the sutures [of the cranium]. See *De usu partium*, Book 9, (K. III: 688; in May's edition, I: 428).

15   Exercise is the next topic.

סבת זה הנחתן ומיעוט התמדתן ואן
התחיל מעט מעט בחדרה אלין
בהתדרגות היה מוצא בסופן מהכח
והחריצות מה שמתחייב להמצא
בסוף כל טיול שרץ על מה שראוי
והואיל וכבר השיב העבד הקטן
על כל פרקי אותן הכתב הנככבד
כמו שצוה הוא מקבץ המלמר
ויקצרהו בפרק אחד יבאר בן
היאך תהיה ההגתאדונע כפי או
המקריס הנמצאיס עתה ואעפ
שזה נתבאר ממה שזכרו העבר
בזן הפרקיס ומה שזכרו כאותו
המאמר אבל הם מזמריס
מפוזריס לא מקובצאס וקורס

1

5

10

15

9: ויקצרהו] Perhaps should read ויאחרהו   11: ואעפ] Abbreviation of ואף על פי.

1 the cause of this is its omission and remission. If he resumes it gradually,
little by little, he will find following it the strength and the vitality that
5 should be found after all exercise that is carried out properly.

Whereas this minor Servant has now responded to all the sections of
that noble letter, as commanded, he will now compile a statement, and
10 follow it with a chapter in which he will make clear what the regimen of
our Master should be, in accordance with those accidents presently occurring. This might well have been made obvious by what this Servant has
mentioned in preceding paragraphs and by what he wrote in that treatise,
15 but these were statements that were dispersed and not properly organized.
Before

Chapter 19

1–5 Training to achieve physical fitness. Maimonides repeatedly mentions the
beneficial influence of physical exercise on health; see, for example, his
Treatise on Asthma, Chapter 5.

6 has now responded: The Latin incunable is discontinued at this point,
probably because the printer felt that this phrase marked the end of the
treatise. The remainder of the text in fact consists of a systematic description
of the regimen recommended for the Sultan, divided into sections dealing
with various foods, or with the program of the day, and supplemented by the
composition of a cardiac remedy taken from Ibn Sina. It ends with a philosophical discourse on medicine and religion.

8 compile: Refers to all the rules of health which he is going to present in the
following statement.

11 presently occurring: The existing symptoms and signs of disease. This demonstrates the cautious medical attitude of Maimonides, who makes pro-
vision for possible changes in the condition of the patient.

1
שאזכור מזה הפרק אומר שהוא ראוי
שיהיה ראוי באוצר אדוננו נוסף
לאותם המנקים שזכרו העבד בפרק
הג׳ מלאמרץ זה קדם שתי מרקחות
5
האחד מהן רפאות מור קרה שכבר
נמוה זקינם שלרפואה שישלהם
זריזות וכראון לה פועל מופלא ע׳
שהם איגם רואים בהפקדרתם זמל׳
משועיה לא נותן אותה ל מאצלם
מרקחת והיא רפאה חברה הראוי
10
בספן בדיחיית הזקנות המזונות:
פרק וזו נוסחותה בלשון מאמרו
להורד הטחון והעבאשיר
והכמפרתא היבשה והכהר בן מכל
אחר חלק ומה לו הקטן חלק מ׳ני
15
ומהמור העוב הטני שמות חלן ויקח

2: ראוי] To be deleted.   3: המנקים] Should read המשקים.   10: הראוי] Should read הראזי.
12: פרק] This indication of a new chapter is missing in the Arabic original. מאמרותיו.

96

1 I begin with this chapter I should say that there ought to be two electuaries
in the treasury of our Master, in addition to those syrups and the Iṭrīfal
which this Servant mentioned in the third chapter of his previous treatise.

5 One of these is a cool musk medicament. The Elders of medicine who
had experience have already tested it, and found it to have an extraordinary
action, so that they do not permit any substitution, or the prescription of
its components separately. Rather, they brought it out as an electuary; it is

10 medicament incorporated by al-Rāzī in his book on the repulsion of the
harm of the nutrients.

This is its description in his very words: There should be taken of pounded
roses, bamboo-manna, dry coriander, and amber, of each, one part; of

15 small pearls, half a part; of the purest and best musk, a sixth of a part.
There should be taken

1–9 The author first suggests that two special medicinal preparations be made
up and kept in the Royal pharmacy. In his treatise *On Poisons*, he makes a
similar suggestion regarding the storage of certain ingredients for preparing
theriac.

4 in his previous treatise: That is, *The Regimen*.

5 musk: For the change of "musk" to "myrrh" in the Hebrew translation, see
the catalogue of plants in this volume, *s.v.* musk (p. 227).

10 The first electuary is taken from the treatise by Rhazes, *On the Repulsion of
the Harm of the Nutrients*. This work is mentioned by Brockelmann, 1937–
1942, I: 420 (38).

14 amber: The Hebrew version uses the Arabic term *kaharaba*. About the
medical uses of amber, see Steinschneider, 1893, p. 701, note 321. He gives
a long quotation in Hebrew from Ibn Sīnā's *De viribus cordis*, in which the
power of attraction of amber is brought into a medical context, thus explaining the "hidden properties" of the mineral substances which Ibn Sīnā
recommends.

מהסובר העברזד ומתירין אותו במי

התפוחין החמוצין השחותין המסועין

ויבושלו עד שיהיה בעמירת הדבש

וימשלי עין בן עליס מעלי האתרוג ולשין

הסמנין בן וירגלזו הרפואה בעל זה

המקרה שהיא רפואה חשובה לחזק

הלב מבלתי חימום ויעיל ללבפקאן

ורפות הלב שעם חמימות

והדפואה הב היא מרקחת

האודים שחברה בן סינא במאמרו

המפורסם ברפואת הלביות וזכר

כמלען ג נוסחאות האחד קר והב חס

והג בינע ומה שרואיהן אדוננו הוא

השוהי וזו עסחת הג פי בלשון מאמרו

אמר הרכבה יאחרת חשובה מאד

עמיתיה מרקחות ואקריא עץ והוספתי

וחסרתי ממעה כפי המזג והיתה

7: ללכפקאן] The inclusion of the second לי is in conformance with the spelling of the Arabic للخفقان.   11: ברפואת] Should read ברפואות.

(*continued from p. 99*)

whom he considered to be suffering from a melancholy disposition. (See Leibowitz, 1970, pp. 52–54). The same disposition is attributed to the Sultan in this treatise. The drugs were prescribed for heart disease as well as for melancholy, which was the main complaint of the Sultan; the jacinth was conceived of as a "sympathetic" drug. See again Steinschneider, 1893, p. 701, note 321.

1   *tabarzad* sugar, dissolved in pressed strained sour apple juice and cooked until it gains the consistence of honey. There should be cast in it leaves of

5   citron, and the medicaments should be kneaded in it. This medicament will take care of one who harbors this accident, for, it is an excellent medicament for strengthening the heart without heating, and it is suitable for palpitation and throbbing of the heart with heat.

10   The second medicament is the jacinth electuary incorporated by Ibn Sīnā in his famous treatise on cardiac remedies; he mentioned three recipes for it, the first cold, the second hot, and the third temperate. The one which this Servant deems suitable for our Master to employ is the temperate, and this is the description of the third in Ibn Sīnā's words:

15   He said: There is another very excellent compound which I have tried as an electuary and in troches, adding to and taking from it according to each and every temperament,

6–8   Here cardiac conditions are mentioned. The indications are: a weak heart, "palpitation," and "throbbing of the heart."

7   without heating: Probably meaning that it would not heat (Arab. *ishan*) the temperament.

8   with heat: Probably in cases with fever (Arab. *harāra*). So far the description of the formula is as given by Rhazes.

9   Now the detailed prescription taken from *De viribus cordis* by Ibn Sīnā begins. The translation of this work into Latin is attributed to Arnold de Villanova (1282 ?). It was appended to several fifteenth century editions of the *Canon*, and also to those of 1527 and 1544, both of which were revised by Andreas Alpagus. There also exist manuscript translations into Hebrew, and we have compared our Hebrew text with the Hebrew manuscripts Munich 280 and 89. For details, see Steinschneider, 1893, pp. 700–701, and Brockelmann, *Suppl.* 1937, I: 827, no. 86. Part of the book has since been translated into English by Gruner, 1930, (pp. 123–125 and 534–552).

10   jacinth: Ruby and other precious stones as well as gold ("aurum potabile") were often used as remedies for heart conditions, more specifically for those compatible with symptoms which would now be classified as coronary artery disease. Previous authors associated melancholy with these cardiac manifestations. As late as 1555, Vesalius, in the second edition of his *Fabrica*, described a parietal thrombus in the left ventricle of the heart, in a patient

(continued on p. 98)

3: אבריסס] Should read אבריסם.   4: ודאנת] Should read ודאנק.   6: הבאדרוג] After this, the equivalent of بزر الباذنجوية is missing.   7: בזמין] Should read בהמן.   11: אסטוכודוס. 12: זראונד] Erroneous translation of جدوار or حدوار.   16–17: דרהם ד' ... תכנגבין is missing in the Arabic text.   16: תכנגבין] Should read סכנגבין or תרנגבין, as in MS Munich 134v 8.

(continued from p. 101)

The first author to attempt to identify the biblical manna as a botanical species was Hiwi al-Balḵi (ninth century). In the comment quoted above, Ibn Ezra rejects Hiwi's identification after examining the plant on his travels in the desert. The modern views have been summarized by A. Kaiser, 1924, and by F. S. Bodenheimer, 1929.

1 and its property of strengthening the heart is highly beneficial. These
are its ingredients: pearls, amber, coral, of each a dram and a half;
shredded silk, burned river crab, of each a miskal and a daniq; ox-
5 tongue, five drams; gold filings, the weight of two daniqs; seeds of
Frankish musk, seeds of sweet basil, and seeds of balm gentle, of each
three drams weight; red behen, white behen, aloe, Armenian stone, washed
lapis lazuli, mastic, bark of cinnamon cassia, cinnamon, saffron, lesser
10 cardamoms of Bawa, big cardamoms, and cubebs, of each a miskal; dodder
of thyme, the weight of two drams and a half; stoechos, the weight of
three drams; zedoary, one miskal, and if not available, then instead of it,
15 zedoary root, two miskals; Greek doronicum, two miskals; seeds of endive,
the weight of five drams; seeds of snake cucumber, the weight of four
drams; manna, the weight of ten drams; red roses, the weight of four drams;

1ff.   Most of these remedies are "sympathetic." According to Ibn Sīnā, they do
not act by their "substance" but only by their "hidden properties," like the
loadstone. (See our running commentary to 143*r*, 4).

1–2   its ingredients: Here the root in Arabic and in Hebrew is equivalent to the
meaning of "leaven." According to Lane, it can be translated: "to put into"
(referring to dough, perfume, wine, and so on). MS. Latin Vienna: "eius
modus." The same root appears on 146*r*, 3, where the translation is "essence."
The Munich MS. 280 is less problematical: "and this is its description."

2   pearls: The Hebrew translation, *bedolaḥ* does not correspond to the modern
usage, in which the term means "crystal." For the biblical usage, see Gesenius,
Dictionary, 1921.

5   gold filings: Ground gold was used as a "sympathetic" drug until the sixteenth century. The Jewish physician Abraham Portaleone published a book
on the medical use of gold in 1584.

9   Cardamom of Bawa: See Meyerhof, 1940, no. 116; called *hīl* (or *hāl*) *buwwa*.
Hāl is still used as a spice added to coffee.

16   in manna: *Tarangubīn*, Meyerhof, 1940, no. 386. In his commentary on
Exodus, 16:13, Abraham Ibn Ezra is opposed to the view that the manna
described in the Bible is identical with "the species used in medicine and
called *tarangubīn*." This opinion is also expressed in the commentary by
Isaac Abrabanel on the same verse. Extensive information on manna is
given by Faber, 1776, Part 2, pp. 81–140.

(continued on p. 100)

מור ב שקלים כאפור שקל עובר שקל   1
סנבל סאדג הנדי מכל אל ב דרהם זהו
העיקר והשאור ולפעמים יושם חלות
ולפעמים תקויבץ בדבש ושתיהן יעשה
כפי המזג השוה ולא ישען ממנו שום   5
דבר ולפעמים ישען למי שיש לו רוע
מזג חם ולמי שיש לו רוע מזג קר
אמנם השוה תונח על ענינה ויושם
מה שקטוף ממנה כל חלה שקל
אג ולשין הכל בשלשת משליהן דבש   10
ואם רצה לחמדה ואחר כך תעשה
עריך שישים בה מהאפיון ה
דרהם ומהגנגד בארסתר שחוק
שחוק כמוהו ולא תעשה לא אחר
שהה חדשים על המעו רצו לומ   15
כשישים בה אפיון ואמנם

.ومن الجندبادستر ومهגדבאדסתר ومهגود باراستر Should read ומהגנד בארסתד 13: .תעשה 11: .ממנו 5:
[אפין 16: .רצוני לומר Abbreviation of [רצו לומֿ 15: Word repeated by mistake. [שחוק 14:
Following this word והגדבאדסתר والجندبادستر is missing.

1 musk, two miskals; camphor, a miskal; ambergris, one miskal; nard and
folia indica, of each, two drams weight; this is the essence. The dough can
be made into troches or combined with honey, and both can be prepared to
5 suit the moderate temperament, which will not be altered, or prepared for
one with a wicked hot temperament, or for one who has an evil cold temperament. As for the moderate, it should be left as it is. When it is to be
made into troches, each troche should be of one miskal. The whole should
10 be kneaded with three parts of honey. If it is desired that it be fermented
and then used, then there must be steeped in it five drams of opium and the
15 same of powdered castoreum. It should not be used except after at least six
months, in case the opium and the castoreum are steeped in it.

3   essence: In the Latin versions this word does not appear, nor does the following word, "dough."

11   fermented: Here the usage is not as in line 3, but refers to actual fermentation.
Opium is more appropriately classified as a "cardiac remedy" than the other
ingredients, and it is still used for coronary heart disease (morphine).

13   Castoreum was regarded by Ibn Sīnā as an antidote to opium; see Francis
Adams, 1847, III: 282, in his commentary on Paulus Aegineta.

מי שגובר עלין רוע מזגחס צריך ~ 1
שישיס כרכומה ומורה חצי שקל
ויחסר ממנה האפיתמון וישיס ~
חילופו ל דרהס שאהתרגוד דרהס
סנא מכיויושס בה הורד משקלי ~ 5
דרהס כסדלחתי ל דרהס ענדלג
דרהס ויונחו הסמנן האחרים בשעס
תקועף כמו שזכרנו ותולש בדבש ~
מוסר הקצף שבער תכלית
ואמנס מי שגובר עלין רוע מזג 10
קר צריך שמוסיפין בסמנן קליפות
אגוז הוא קליפות האתרוג על הבלסאן
זנגביל פלפל מכלא משקל דרהס
שע שקליס ומספיק לו מהכאפור
חצי שקל ויספיק לבעל המזג החס 15
יקח חצי השתיה ממנה עס שקל

5: י.   6: דרהם] Following this, the words זרע בקלא המקא שמונה דרהם טבאשיר חמשה זרע חזרת (according to the Arabic text as well as to the translation in MS. Munich 134v 19-20) are missing. בסד אלחתי] In the Arabic Mss.: Cod. Uri 555 بزر الحبشى , Poc. 280 (Neubauer 1270[5]) אלקתי; Hebr. translation in Ms. Munich חזרת.   12: הוא] Should read בוא.   16: חצי השתיה.

1   For one who is dominated by a bad hot temperament, reduce the saffron and the musk to half a miskal, omit the dodder of thyme, and use in its
5   stead five drams of fumitory and four drams of senna of Mecca. Steep in it roses, ten drams weight; seeds of purslane, eight drams; bamboo-manna, five drams; seeds of asphodel, two drams; and sandalwood, three drams. The other ingredients should be kept as they are. It should be made into troches as we have mentioned, and kneaded with honey, thoroughly skimmed of its foam.

10   For one who is dominated by a bad cold temperament, add to the medicaments nutmeg rind, citron rind, balsam wood, ginger and pepper, of each a dram weight, and castoreum, two miskals; the camphor should be restricted to half a miskal.

15   Whoever has a hot temperament should proceed to take half a draught of this with a miskal

3   omit the dodder of thyme: As not suitable for the "hot temperament." Maimonides classified *Cuscuta epithymum* under drugs which are "hot and dry" (*Aphorisms*, XXI).

6   senna of Mecca: Following this, the Hebrew translator has omitted a number of the ingredients, some of which are retained in MSS. Hebrew Munich 280 and 87.

14   two miskal: Before this, the word "castoreum" is missing in the Jerusalem manuscript but occurs in MSS. Hebrew Munich 280 and 87, which are translations of Ibn-Sīnā's *De viribus cordis*.

ובאשיר בדבש התפוחין ובעל המזג   1

הקר יקח ממנה עם משקל טסונן

וכבר רפאתי קצתמי שרץ ריעת

המלכיס מכאב קשה נועה למאינה

והוספתי בנוסחא השוה משקל חצי   5

דרהם אורם שחוק הדיק והיה רמוע

חשוב והועלן תועלת חזקה אחר

היאוש · ואמנס ההרכבה

המיוחדת לבעלי המזגם החמין

שיקרה להם הקפלאן וחלישות   10

הלב לסבת רוע מזגם החם יש

ממנה הרכבה בזו הנוסח זרע

החזרת זרע האפאחיס זרע הקרא

זרע היקשואיס קלופים מכל אחד

משקל ה' דרהם זרע עירק השוה   15

2: טסונן] Following this word גדבאדסתר is missing.   4: למאינה] Should read למאניה.
10: הקפכאן] Should read הקפקאן   الخفقان הח׳פקאן   13: הקרא] Should read הקרע according to the
Arabic spelling القرع.

(continued from p. 107)

wild animals." The Paris manuscript has: "from the severe pain, this is
total madness." However MSS. Poc. and Hunt. have: "wild madness" (rage).

10   palpitation [= syncope] and weakness of the heart: These syndromes follow
immediately after the discussion of melancholia. Heart disease, especially of
coronary origin, is often attended by fear and a sensation of impending death.
palpitation: *Khafaqān* in Arabic and *qafakan* in our Hebrew manuscript is
translated in the Latin *Canon* of Ibn Sīnā as "passio cardiaca," a term introduced by Caelius Aurelianus (see Leibowitz, 1970, p. 37).

1 of bamboo-manna in apple rob. He who harbors a cold temperament
should take a draught of it with one-twelfth of a dram weight of castoreum.

I have already treated some of those who follow the same course as kings
suffering from melancholia, a disorder that tends toward mania, that is
5 rage. In these cases, I added to the temperate recipe the weight of dram of
thoroughly pulverized jacinth, of exquisite pomegranate color, and they
were greatly benefited by it, after previous despair.

As to the compound specific for those who harbor a hot temperament,
10 and are attacked by palpitation and weakness of the heart because of the
badness of their hot temperament, there is a composition of this description:
lettuce seeds, melon seeds, pumpkin seeds, and shelled snake-cucumber
15 seeds, of each five drams weight; purslane seeds,

3–4 who follow the course: Of manic-depressive disease, in which phases of
melancholia alternate with maniacal excitement. The author was aware of
the course of this mental disease, which was only fully described in the
nineteenth century.

4 kings: This appears to mean that he had already treated other persons of
high rank who were suffering from melancholy, as was his princely patient
to whom this treatise applies; an encouraging remark by the author.

It is also possible that Maimonides is here alluding to the idea that kings
and other leaders are especially prone to melancholy. This notion may be
traced to the Pseudo-Aristotelian *Problemata*, Book XXX, 953a, 10 ff.,
translation by W. S. Hett: "Why is it that all men who have become outstanding in philosophy, statesmanship, poetry, or the arts are melancholic,
etc."? See the work of Klibansky *et al. Saturn and Melancholy*, 1964, in
which the philosophical, historical and medical implications have been
discussed. A similar belief was expressed, for example, by Adam of Fulda
in his book on music (1490); he refers to King Saul's attack of "melancholy"
as a condition which predominantly affects "kings, princes, and rulers."
This he attributes, however, to "the burden of their responsibilities." (See
Kümmel, 1969.) The term "royal disease" occurs in Latin with reference to
another condition, icterus: see the Latin translations of the *Aphorisms* of
Hippocrates (V, 71); Celsus, III: 24 (p. 338 in the Loeb edition); Castellus,
1746, p. 413: "icterus, alias Morbus Regius."

mania, that is rage: The last words are missing in the Jerusalem Hebrew
MS. They are, however, retained in the Munich manuscript: "madness of

(*continued on p. 106*)

משקל ג דרהם כרולח כסד כהרכא   1
סרטן נהריי שרוף מֵשי מקוצץ מכל
א שקל דבש הכדר שקל ואם לא ימצא
יושם עץ הכדר ג משקליס עץ ~
הגרי צרוג זדנכאד כהמן לכן מן   5
כל אחד ב דרהס טפאשיר קענה ־
מכל א ג דרהס ורד אדוס מוסר
מיובש בכל משקלן דרהס כרמס
חצי שקל שחוק עד שכשה מור ~
שחיקה חזקה וסכשה ענבר מהכל   10
משקל שקל וחצי לשון שור ה שקלס
כל זה כמ שביא והלישה במי התפוחין
ודבש החבושים ודבש הרמונס כד
בכד כשיעור מה שלשין אותה ־
והמצע גולאבי וקח כשחיטת לשון שור   15

5: [צרונג Should read דרונג' درونج   6: [טבאשיר Following this word, قاله قاקלה
is missing.   9: [שקל Following this word, كافور כאפור is missing. [סכשה Scribe's mistake;
should read כעשיריתו (according to MS. Munich 135r 19).   10: [וסכשה See above;
should read שביארנו   [שביא Abbreviation of   [כמ 12: Abbreviation of כמו.   ושישיתו should read.

1 the weight of four drams; pearls, coral, amber, burned river crab, and
shredded silk, of each a miskal; rob of pandanus palm, a miskal, and if
that is not available, wood of the pandanus palm, three miskals; aloes,
5 doronicum, zedoary, and white behen, of each two drams weight; red roses
plucked from the stalk and dried in the shade, seven drams weight; saffron,
10 half a miskal; camphor with a tenth of its weight of thoroughly pulverized
musk, and a sixth of ambergris, of the whole, one and a half miskal; oxtongue, five miskals. The whole of this should be made into troches as we
have explained, or kneaded in rob of apple, rob of quince or rob of pomegranate in parts equal to that in which it is kneaded.
15   There is also a julep of the above. It is taken with the expressed juice of
oxtongue

2   burned river crab: Cf. *Picatrix*, (1962, p. 410, note 2): "ashes of a sea crab."
River crab is recommended in the Hebrew *Book of Experiences* attributed to
Abraham Ibn Ezra, which exists only in manuscript form.

shredded silk: According to Ibn al-Bayṭār, this possesses the properties of
"cheering the heart," activating the vital forces, and improving the mental
faculties and the memory.

7   plucked from the stalk: In the Hebrew text, "removed"; in the Arabic,
"from which the stalks have been removed."

עם כמוהו סחיטת העולשין וג' כמוהו
סחיטת התפוחים וכמו הכל פעמים
מי הורד ושתות מה שנתקן כן סוכר
עכ'זד ויבושל בנחת עד שיתבשל
והגולאב הנלקח בעלי הבאדרנביה
מבושל במי הורד עד שיקח כח ואן
תרשם סחיתתן במי הורד שליש ורב
שלישים מועיל לכל מי שיש לו חלישות
הלב ובלבד אם היה עמן לשון שור
אמנם היבש יבושל עמן במי הורד
ואמנם הלח יומזג בשחיתתן ואם
היה המזג **חזק** החמי מות ממעין
הכדרנגם ויוסף בסחיתת לשון
השור ואם לא חלקים שוים וראו'גל
שאזכור מעני המזונות שיוקחו תמיד

5: הבאדרנבויה] Should read הבאדרנג'ויה الۡبادرنجوية .   12: ממעין] Following this word,
بادرنجوية .   13: הכדרנגם] Scribe's error; should be transcription of
סחיטת عصارة is missing.

1 with an equal quantity of expressed juice of endive, four times its quantity
of apple juice, twice the whole of rose water, and a sixth of the whole of
5 *tabarzad* sugar; it should be cooked gently until thickened. This julep,
taken with leaves of balm gentle cooked in rose water until it gains its
virtues, or with balm gentle juice diluted in rose water one-third to two-
thirds, is beneficial to all those who have a weakness of the heart, especially
10 if it contains oxtongue which, if dry, should be cooked with it in rose
water, and if fresh, should be mixed with its expressed juice. If the temperament is intensely hot, reduce the juice of balm gentle and increase the juice
of oxtongue; otherwise, they should be taken in equal quantities.
15   I should mention also the preparation of the nutriments which are usually   Chapter 20
taken.

4 tabarzad sugar: *albissimo succaro* in the Latin translation of *De viribus cordis*, from which the whole recipe was taken.

5 leaves of balm gentle: See Meyerhof, 1940, no. 40.

14 in equal quantities: This is the end of the quotation from Ibn Sīnā's *De viribus cordis*, which we have compared with MS. Hebrew Munich 280, as well as with the Latin edition.

ותחלתם הלחם משתדלין בטוב ~

החטה ולא יעשה סולת נקיה ר'ל

אין מטבילין אותה במים כמן שהוא

המנהג אבל ממרי־צין לכברו עד

שלא ישאר בן שום דבר מהמורסן

וממרי־צין בלישתן ויהיה ע־יה־

המלח ראה השאור ויהין החלות

חסרי התוך ואופין אותן בתנור־

או בפורע והתנור יותר עוב׃

הכשר מכונן שיהיה כשר תרעגלות

או תרנגלין ושומן המרק שלהם

תמיד שזה המין מהעוף יש לו סגלה

בהתקנת הלחות המופסדות.אי זה

פסידות שיהיה ובלבד הלחות

השחורות עד שהרופאים אמרו

2: [ר'ל] **Abbreviation of** רוצה לומר.   4: [לכברו] **Should read** לכברו.

1 Their first is bread, which is the goodness of the wheat. It should not be made white; by that I mean that it should not be immersed in water as the
5 custom goes, and it should not be sifted thoroughly until none of the bran remains in it. It should be kneaded exceedingly well, and it should be noticeably salty and well raised. The loaves should have no crumb, and it should be baked in the circular earthen oven, or in any oven; the earthen oven is better.
10 *The Meat:* As far as possible, the meat should be that of hens or roosters and their broth should also be taken, because this sort of fowl has virtue in rectifying corrupted humors, whatever the corruption may be, and
15 especially the black humors, so much so that the physicians have mentioned

4   should not be sifted thoroughly: The translation into English amends the text by adding the negative ("not to be sifted"), in order to agree with the directions given by Maimonides in the first chapter of his *Regimen* (Bar-Sela's edition, p. 18). However, a change of mind on the part of Maimonides may also be implied. Indeed, there are a number of instances of such deviations in his views, even in purely legal decisions. In the same way, scholars have found inconsistencies in the views expressed by Galen, whom Maimonides studied assiduously and tried to emulate. Galen's changing opinions have been demonstrated in a paper, "On Translating Galen," by Margaret T. May, 1970. In fact, all the Arabic manuscripts of our treatise recommend sifting the wheat. See our medical contents (p. 28), in which we quote parallels to Galen's view that coarse bread has lesser nutritional value and is more rapidly excreted by the bowel, especially, *De alimentorum facultatibus*, I, 2, (K. VI: 480 ff.). Here Maimonides advocates separation of the bran, but the ultimate condition of the flour should not be too refined. He seems to follow Galen's statement: "Between bread made very white and that which is very coarse there exists a quite wide range of more or less."

11–14 broth: Meat extracts exert a beneficial effect on the mucous membrane of the stomach in those cases of gastritis which are accompanied by a low level of gastric acidity.

113

שהמרק של תרנגלות מועיל מהרתן   1

ולא יוקח מזה המין לא גדול שפאן

עלין שותים ולא קטנן שהדיר עלין

גובר ולא הכחוש ממנו ולא מה

שמשמנן אותו ביד אלא השמן ממנו   5

שאינן אבוס וצורת הנהגתו כך

שמתירין התרנגולת והתרנגולין

בחרבה רחבה לא יהיה בה ולא

לכלוך ומבקרין לנקותה ולכברה

תמיד ויותן להם המאכל שאוכלין   10

אותו בראשי היומם בכלים ויהא

קמח שעורים מולש בחלב חלוב

ואם חותכו התאנים היבשים וערב

עמו יהיה יותר משובח ולא ינשם

להן מהמאכל כי אם מלא זפקיהם   15

בלבד ויונח להם מים אחר שעות

2: נדולו] Abbreviation of גדולות.   3: שותים] Should read שנתים.   8: בה] Following this, the equivalent of مزبلة מזבלה is missing.   15: זפקיהם.

1 that chicken broth is beneficial in leprosy. Of this species, neither the old which has attained two years should be taken, not the young in which
5 mucus is predominant, not the weak, not those force-fed, but rather the fattest among those that are not stall-fed.

    The manner of their management is as follows: The hens and roosters
10 should be let loose in spacious ruins, wherein there is no dunghill or dirt, tended with cleanliness and constant sweeping. The food that they eat should be placed before them at the beginning of the day in vessels; it should be barley flour kneaded in fresh milk. It is even better if dried figs are
15 chopped and mixed with it. Food should be given to them only in an amount that fills their crops. Water should be given to them. After several hours,

1   that chicken broth is beneficial in leprosy: See the German translation by Richter, 1910, of 'Alī b. al-'Abbās (tenth century) on leprosy, especially pp. 325–326. The disease is there attributed to a dry temperament and to the predominance of black bile. Maimonides recommends chicken broth, which was presumed to exert a good effect on the atrabilis.

6   nor those force-fed: See *Babylonian Talmud*, Tractate *Baba Meẓi'a*, 86v, where Samuel, the physician, recommends fowl and oxen which are naturally fat and not force-fed.

8   ruins: Kroner's translation is "Kasten oder Verschlag." Both translations are acceptable according to the reading of the diacritical points of the Arabic text. The word "dunghill" is missing in the Hebrew Ms.

9   cleanliness: In order to avoid contamination.

10–16 Food should be given: Attention is paid to a special "formula." The influence of animal feed, in this case with reference to milk production, is noted by Galen in *De sanitate tuenda*, p. 210 of the English translation by Green, 1951. See also the *Canon* of Ibn Sīnā, Book 1, Fen 3, Chapter 2.

שוען להם חיטים נשורין במים שעות   1
ובסוף היום מביאין לפניהם גם כן ~
קמח שעורין ותאנים מחותכין מולשן
בחלב והתר נעלות והתר נוגלין ~
שמהיגין אותם חלבם לבן מערן   5
ומתבשל בזמן יותר מהרה ומרעב
המזג מאד נמשורה אותן וככבר
נתאמתו לו הדבריים ונתבארה
תועלתם ואם ישנא להתמיד מקצ א
אין רוע שיוקח בקצתה הימים   10
אבל התוריס יש בהן יבשות ואעף
שיש להם סגולה נפלאה בהטרת
השכל וכמו כן הקורא אינ רואה
לאדונינו בן מפני שהוא מאמץ בן
מעיס ואם עתאותה הנפש לכשר   15
הבהמות יהיה כשר גדי יונק ·

1 wheat should be scattered before them after soaking it for hours in water.
At the end of the day, barley flour and chopped figs kneaded with milk
5 should again be put before them. In hens and roosters thus managed, we
find the suet white and delicious; it cooks as rapidly as possible, moistens
the temperament greatly and renders it moderate. These things have already
been tested, and their value is manifest.

10   Should repetition of the same variety become tedious, there is no harm
in taking instead on some days, francolin or grouse. As to the turtle dove,
there is dryness in it, although it has a unique virtue in kindling the mind.
I do not deem the partridge suitable for our Master because it causes
15 retention of stools.

    If the spirit craves the meat of cattle, it should be that of a suckling kid.

7   renders it moderate: Moderation of the temperament was regarded as the
goal of health measures, and dyscrasia was thought of as leading to disease,
even to leprosy, as assumed by 'Alī b. al-'Abbās (see the note to line 1, 149*r*).

8   tested: The validity of empirical verification was often stressed in medieval
medicine.

12–13 kindling the mind: In Arabic "sharpening the intellect," in Hebrew "puri-
fying the intellect." This appears to be an overestimate of the effect of diet
on mental capacity.

ואם אי אפשר על כל פנים מבשר הכבש   1
לוקחין מהטלאים מה שלא נשלמה לו
שנה · ויקח מבשר המוקדם נדבר
ולא יהיה שמן הרבה לאמן הרועים אלת
ולא יוקח שום דבר לא אם שנא מהתרע   5
והתרנגלין   היוך יכין ממנו ·
הלכן הנראה מה שאפשר הדק ·
העמדה הטוב הטעם ואם היה בו
עפיצות ותעיין רוע הריח שעברה
עליו שנה אחר או קרוב ולה ויזהר   10
מחזק האדמומית והעב·
בעמדי או המשונה בריח או היין
ולזה המרירות לא יקרב לשום·
דמי מלו המינם בשום פנים · ש
התבשילים נושים להיות התבשילין   15
מתוקי הטעם או יהיה להם חמצות
מועטות ·   והנע אזכור תבשילין ·

1 If there is no avoiding, at times, the meat of sheep, those lambs that have not attained a year, but approach it, should be chosen. The forepart of the meat, especially, should be taken; it should not be excessively fat, but from
5 grazing animals. Nothing of these should be taken unless hens or roosters become wearisome.

The Wine: One should take that which is as white in color as possible, of fine essence, of good taste—and if there is a little astringency in it, there is
10 no harm—of good odor and that which has aged for a year or close to it. Beware of that which is intensely red, or thick of essence, or altered in odor, or old and intensely bitter; one should not approach anything of these kinds at all.

15 *The Dishes:* As far as possible, the dishes should be sweet in taste or have in them a little or just perceptible sourness. I shall herewith mention a number of dishes,

3 The forepart of the meat: This part is known to possess a lesser fat content. Maimonides was opposed to the inclusion of much fat in the diet; this was one of his most cherished medical precepts (see *Hilkot de'ot,* 4:15; *Aphorisms,* IX). It would accord with modern views on the subject of animal fat.

7–8 of fine essence: For "essence" our Hebrew translation uses the word *'emdah* and the Berlin manuscript uses *'ezem,* meaning the body (of the wine) and denoting a fluid or cohesive property as found, for example, in burgundy or in its counterpart, malaga.

9 astringency: A property of medicinal use, because it stimulates gastric acidity and counteracts catarrhal manifestations.

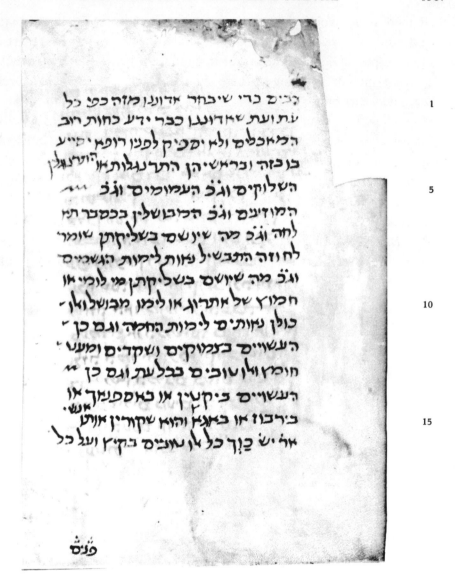

רבים כדי שיבחר אדוענ ומזה כפי כל
עת ועת שאדוענ כבר ידע כחות רוב
המאכלם ולא יספיק לפני רופא יסיע
בו כזה ובראשיהן התרנגלותא והירנולן
השלוקים וגב העמומים וגב
המוזיעם וגב המבושלין בכמבר תי
לח וגב מה שינשם בשליקתן שומר
לח וזה התבשיל נאות לימות הגשמיים
וגב מה שינשם בשליקתן מי לימי או
חמוץ של אתרוג או לימן מבושלוגן
כולן נאותים לימות החמה וגם כן
העשויים בצמוקים ושקדים ומעט
חומץ ולו עובים בבלעת וגם כן
העשויים בקטין או באספנך או
בירבוז או באגצ והוא שקורין אותו אנש
אלו יש כוך כל און נועבים בקיץ ועל כל

פّנّס

1: רבים.   5: וגב] Abbreviation of וגם כן.   6: המוזעים.   15: באגאצ.   16: אר יש] Abbreviation of אר יש] Abbreviation אר ישׁ] ארץ ישראל of.

1   so that our Master may choose from them those appropriate for each and
every occasion, because our Master already knows the virtues of most of
the foods, and a physician will not fail to be at hand to be relied upon in
this regard.

5   The first is hens or roosters, boiled or broiled in a pit, or steamed, or
cooked with chervil, or cooked in water into which green fennel is cast;
these dishes are suitable in the winter time. Those cooked in water to
10   which lemon juice, cedrat pulp or mixed lemons are added, are suitable in
the summer time. Those prepared with almonds, sugar, lemon juice and
wine are suitable in every season. Those prepared with currants, almonds,
and a little vinegar are excellent at any time. Those prepared in *Isfidbaj*
with beets or lettuce in the summertime and those prepared with round
15   pumpkins, or spinach, or blite, or with prunes, which the people of Syria
call *Khawkh*, are all good in the summer.

3   a physician will not fail to be at hand: Although paying tribute to the Sultan's own knowledge of dietetics, the author notes that a physician should
be consulted when special problems arise.

4–16   The preparation of the dishes differs according to the season of the year.
The author maintains that certain vegetables and fruits should be added to
meat dishes, presumably on account of their nutritive properties.

9–10   lemon juice: The citrus fruits which he recommends ("cedrat pulp," line 10)
are particularly rich in vitamin C.

11–13   In the Hebrew text, following line 11 a sentence is missing, and following
line 13 a few of the ingredients have been changed.

16   Syria: In the Hebrew text this is rendered "Land of Israel."

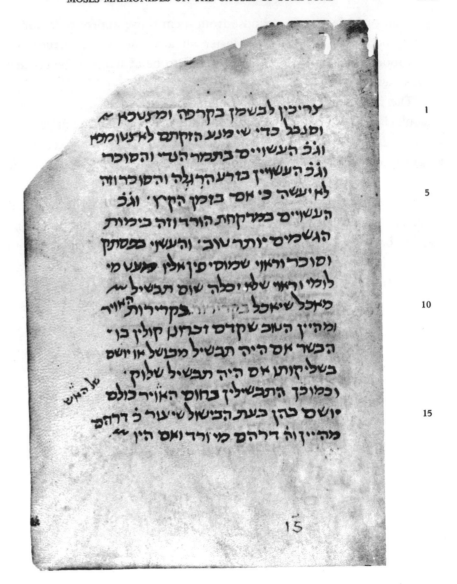

עריכין לבשמן בקרפה ומעטכאן ~

וסנבל כדי שי מנע הזקתם לארעו/מס

וגכ העשוייס בתמר הכדי והסוכר

וגכ העשויין בורע הרגלה והסוכר וזה

לאיעשה כי אסי בזמן היקץ · וגכ

העשויים במריקחת הורד וזה בימות

הגשמיס יותר טוב· והעשיי מסתן

וסוכר וראוי שמוסי סין ואלן מעט מי

לומי וראוי שלא יכלה שוס תבשיל ~

מאכל שיאכל בקרירות . בקרירות האויר

ומהיין הטוב שקדס וכרנו קולין בן ·

הכשר אס היה תבשיל מבושל או יושם

בשליקותן אם היה תבשיל שלוק ·

וכמוכן התבשילין כחוס האויר כולם

יושס כהן כעת הבישול שיעור כ דרהם

מהיינה דרהם מי ורד ואס הין ~

10: שיאכל] After this, the first word of the erroneously doubled בקרירות has been erased.
14: האויר] Marginal note by a later hand של האש.

1 One should not neglect spicing them with cinnamon bark, mastic, and nard to prevent any harm to the stomach. Those prepared with tamarind and sugar, and those prepared with purslane seeds and sugar, should not be
5 used except in the summer, while those prepared with rose preserves are better in the winter. The one prepared with pistachio and sugar ought to have a little lemon juice added to it.
10 The dish of food eaten in cool weather should not lack the good drink, described previously. The meat should be fried in it, if it is a cooked dish, or it should be added to the soup, if it is a boiled dish. Likewise, during
15 warmer weather there should be added to all the dishes during cooking a measure of twenty drams of wine and five drams of rose water; if the dishes are

1 One should not neglect spicing them: Here the reason for the use of spices is quite explicit, because the sentence closes with the words: "to prevent any harm to the stomach." On the therapeutic use of spices see the note by Schedel, 1919. The physiological action of spices on gastric secretion was noted by Pavlov, 1897, Chap. 8. It is possible that the addition of spices and wine was also thought to prevent spoilage of the food.

11 in it: Meaning the electuary described above.

fried: The Hebrew term is *ḳolin*, meaning to roast, but in this case the term "pot roast" should be used, because the meat was cooked in the liquid electuary and no fat is mentioned. It is noteworthy that the suggested methods of cooking are fat-free, in accordance with the author's dietetic principles mentioned above.

1

התבשילין חמוצים יהיה מהיין כ׳ דהם
 נממי הורד חמשה נממי הלימון ק׳ נג׳
התרנגלות צלויות על השפוד על המנהג
נאשקין אותן תמיד בשעת צלייתן בין
ומי הלימו ובין לבדו ואם קצה הנפש ~

5

לעליית בשר השפדים יהיה יונק אחר
משיחתו כשרתמרצעה צליה בין למעט
כרכום וכל מאכל שיתבן לשים בן מעט
כרכום לפי שהוא רפאה לבית המשמח
ולא ירבה ממנו שהוא ישלו סגולה ___

10

בהפלת תאותה מאכל וזה מה שנזכר
העבד עתה מתבשילי המאכל ~
שראויים לאדוננן יתמיד הא ימין ·
נכבר זכר גאינום נמי שקדכון מהרופאי

15

משקה קורין אותם כלשועם אדרומא
נהין עושין אותו מדבש דבוריס יין לבן
דק כמו שהיו עושין הסכנגבין מסוכר

14: מהרופאי] Abbreviation for מהרופאים.

(*continued from p. 125*)

17 sugar: A still later addition. Here the author displays his historical sense
when he describes the successive changes in the composition of a time-honored
drug.

oxymel: Another preparation used since antiquity. To the orginal formula of
vinegar and honey, many ingredients were added over the ages: see Galen
(K. XVIII B: 466) in his *Commentary on Hippocrates on Fractures*, Book II.

For other varieties of this drink, in which roses or currants were added,
see below, 155*v*, 5–6.

1   to be sour, there should be added twenty drams of the wine, five of rose
water, and five of lemon juice. If it is a chicken, broiled on a spit as is
5   customary, it should be basted while roasting with wine and lemon juice,
or wine alone.

If the spirit craves roast meat of cattle, it should be the suckling kid,
basted while roasting with wine and a little saffron. To each meal, a little
saffron should be added, because it is a cheering cardiac medicament; it
10 should not be in excess, because it has the property of quieting the appetite
for food.

This is what this Servant now presents on the dishes of food which suit
our Master, may his days be prolonged.

Galen, and those who preceded him among the physicians, mentioned a
15 drink which they name in their language *hydromel;* they used to prepare it
from honey and thin white wine, as they used to prepare oxymel from
vinegar

6   meat of cattle: The Hebrew text here uses the word *shepudim* ("spits")
figuratively for the Arabic term for quadrupeds, because beef (meat of
cattle) was usually roasted on a spit.

8   saffron: Was thought to affect both the heart and the emotions.
The term *karkum* in Semitic languages is used for two different plant products:
saffron (*Crocus sativus*) and turmeric (*Curcuma longa L.*). See Löw, II: 7 ff.

11 appetite: The author mentions the adverse effect on the appetite; it was
usual with him to consider the side effects.

14 who preceded him: Hydromel was one of the drugs most often prescribed
by Hippocrates. However, he does not appear to have noted its property of
"dilating the spirit" (152*r*, 4).
Galen rarely uses the term "hydromel," but rather *melikraton* (*De alimentorum facultatibus*, Book III, Chapter 39; K. VI: 741, and elsewhere), as in
older Greek literature including the Odyssey. Wherever the term "hydromel"
is used in the Jones translation of Hippocrates, the original Greek term is
melikraton (see *Regimen in Acute Diseases*, Jones edition II, Chapter 12 and
elsewhere). See also Dierbach, 1824, p. 76.

16 and thin white wine: The original hydromel was prepared from water and
honey. However, Maimonides mentions the later addition of wine.

(continued on p. 124)

וחומץ כך עשו האדרומלי מסוכרויין 1
וזה משקה משובח מאד לחיזוק ~
האצטומכא והלב וליפות העיכול ~
והרחבת הנפש ומסייע על רעיאת שע ~
היתרונות פינע טוב נסיכן זה ונסהן 5
זולתגן פעמים רבות ונוסח עשיתן ~
שיוקח מהסוכר ה' רוטלים מצרייס
ומבשלין אותו כמו שמבשלין המשקים
ומסיריו קצפו ויוקח לו בישול טוב ואחר
זה יושם עליו רוטל אחד במצרי מהיין 10
הנזכר ויבושל משקה בעמדת משקה
שלורד ולא יזכר העבד זה המשקה
עס המאכלים כי אם מפני שהארץ
יוקח תמיד בכלינס כראשי היומסי
בימות הגשמים במים חמין ובימות 15
הקיץ במים קריס ויוקח ממנו ג אוקיו
וד' אוקיאות בפעם אחת שזה משקה

10: עליו] Following this, יין is added by a later hand.   16: אוקיו] Abbreviation for אוקיות.
17: אוקיאות] Should read אוקיות.

1 and honey. But their successors, as they prepared oxymel from sugar and vinegar, prepared hydromel from sugar and wine. This is a most excellent drink, beneficial in strengthening the stomach and the heart, improving the 5 digestion, dilating the spirit, and easing the egress of the two superfluities with good effect. We have tested it, as have others, time and again.

The description of its preparation is: take five Egyptian pounds of sugar, cook it as syrups are cooked, removing its foam, until it acquires a good 10 consistency. Then cast into it one Egyptian pound of good wine, and thicken it into a syrup of the consistency of syrup of roses. This Servant has mentioned this syrup along with the foods only because it resembles them. It should always be taken daily at the beginning of the day, in the wintertime in hot water and in the summertime in cold water. Three or 15 four ounces should be taken at a time, because this syrup

4–5 egress of the two superfluities: Metabolic end-products eliminated in the feces and urine. See our introduction, p. 15, and medical contents, p. 30.

5 tested: Here again Maimonides lays stress on repeated evaluation of the efficacy of drugs (see 149*v*, 8).

7 pound: The Hebrew text says *rotl* which is similar to the Arabic term; this is a transposition of the letters of the word *litra*. The latter form appears in the Berlin manuscript.

9 removing its foam: See Galen on oxymel preparations, *De sanitate tuenda*, Book IV, Chapter 6 (K. VI: 271–274): Honey is boiled with water, the froth is removed, and vinegar is added. Removal of the froth is also mentioned by Donnolo (tenth century), but with regard to herbal potions containing honey. See Leveen, 1927–1928.

consistency: As in the Berlin MS. (*'aẓmut*). The Jerusalem Hebrew MS. gives *bishūl*, but with the same meaning.

13 resembles: In Hebrew *raẓ*, literally "runs as," that is, "resembles" food. For a different meaning of *raẓ*—"runs," as the "course" of a disease, see 147*r*, 3.

127

אינו משקה הטבנזמין וחולתן מהדומה [ן
שאותם המשקים מזון משובח שהסוכר
במופרדו מזון ואעפ שיש בן רפואותית
מועטת וכמו כן היין משובח מזון כל ~
ספק יותר פלא מה שאמרו שהוא אינו ~
מזיק לחמי המזג ואין סבתזה אלא היות
פשוטין מזונות.   פרק כהסדרת
ההנהגה כפי מה שק כל אדונגן יסיר
הא כהבן ויתמיד ימין ואין ספק שזה
המאמר יגע לאדונגנ כבוא הגשמיס
לפי ראה העבר שיתחיל כערת ~
ההנהגה שיתנהג בה בקור האויר
והעבר מיחל שאדונגנ כשיתמיד זו
ההנהגה תחזור בריאותן להדגל ~
ביותר מהר אם ירצה הא ית. והעבד
אינו יודע מנהג אדונגן כעת הבריאות
אם הוא אוכל פעם אחת או מזון בבקר.

1 is not like the syrup of oxymel and others of its kind, since those drinks are medicaments requiring apportioning and discernment regarding whom they suit, while this drink is an excellent nutriment because the sugar alone is a nutriment, although it is only slightly medicative, and the wine is also an

5 excellent nutrient, without any doubt. What is most admirable about it, it is said, is that it does not harm the choleric, and the reason for this is simply that its ingredients are familiar good nutriments.

10 This is the measure of what this Servant has envisaged presenting before mentioning the order of the regimen.

Chapter 21

On the management of a regimen for our Master in accordance with his complaints — may God remove his pains and perpetuate his days.

There is no doubt that this tract will reach our Master at the approach of winter, and therefore this Servant thought he should begin with the kind of regimen which he should follow in cold weather. This Servant hopes that, if our Master perseveres in this regimen, his health will return to normal in

15 as short a time as God the Most High may will. This Servant does not know the habits of our Master in the state of health, whether he eats but once a day or whether he takes breakfast and supper.

1 like the syrup: The word "like" is missing in our Hebrew manuscript but is correctly inserted in Hebrew MS. Berlin.
syrup: The Arabic and Hebrew terms denote "drink." The Hebrew transliteration of *sakanǧubīn* (oxymel) is here corrupted, but is correctly written on 151ν, 17 and on 155ν, 5. Following the first line, a phrase in the Hebrew text is missing, but it appears in the Berlin fragment.

2–3 nutriment . . . medicative: On nutrients and medicaments, see our medical contents, pp. 24 and 30.

5 doubt: In the Hebrew manuscript, a full stop is missing after this word.

7 A few words are missing from this line in the Hebrew text.
Here begins Chapter 21, dealing with the regimen in general.

7–17 With regard to mealtimes, the author refers to the custom of eating only one or two meals a day. A similar habit is referred to in Exodus 16:12.

10 winter: In Arabic and Hebrew, "rainy season," that is, winter.

17 breakfast: Delete full stop following this word in the Hebrew text.

ובערב לפ' ינהיג ההנהגה כפי ב' ענינם

ואומר יכוין שתהיה הה יערה מהשיעה

לעולם עם צאת השמש או קודם זה

במעט ויוקחו אז ממשקה אדרומלי ב

אוקיאות או ג'וי מתן אחר זה שעה י'רב

ולא יסורם ירכב בלאט ובכה תדרגות

במהירות התנועה עד שיתחממו

האברים ותשתנה הנשימה אז ירד

וינוח עד שלו ישאר במישוש הגש

והנשימה שום דבר ממה שנשהן

הטיול ואחר זה יזון בא מן התבשילין

שהדם זכרונם ויקח מעט מהפירות

המאמצים כמו שכבר נאמר או גרעיני

פיסתק וצמוקים או מעט מהמתיקה

היבושה או מעט מרקחת שלורד כל

זה כפי מה שהרגילו עתה אחר זה יסב

1

5

10

15

1: לפי] Abbreviation ot *Abbreviation of* 2: לפי זה. ההערה 11: בא] *Abbreviation of* באחד.

130

1 On this account, he will mention the regimen appropriate for both conditions.

I declare that one should always aim to awaken from sleep at sunrise or
5 a little before that. Two or three ounces of the syrup of hydromel should
be taken at that time. He should wait thereafter for an hour and then go
riding. He should ride leisurely, and then, without stopping, gradually
quicken the pace until the members are warmed and the respiration alters.
Then he should dismount, and rest until none of the changes caused by
10 exercise remain on the skin of the body or in the respiration. After that, he
should partake of one of the dishes mentioned previously. He should take
some of the astringent fruits as has already been said, or kernels of pistachio
and currants, or a little of the dry sweetmeats, or a little of rose preserves,
15 depending upon what he is now using. Then he should recline

1   mention: The Hebrew text uses the word for "outline."

3   at sunrise: This refers to the winter, when the sun rises late. The regimen for
the summer begins on 155v, 3.

4   syrup of hydromel: Probably to promote the evacuations ("egress of the two
superfluities," 154r, 4–5).

5   riding: Sport held an important place in the medical system of the author.
In his medical *Aphorisms*, he devotes the whole of Section 18 to physical
exercise.

7–8   Refers to physiological changes brought about by exercise; see our medical
contents, p. 30.

11   dishes: This indicates quite a substantial breakfast (see 150v ff.), which seems
to have been the main meal of the day.

13   as has already been said: See 140r, 3–7, which refers to the use of astringent
fruits after taking "whatever softens the stools."

15   rose: Dierbach, 1824, classifies roses among the astringent substances mentioned by Hippocrates.

לשעה וינגן המנגן ביתר ויגביה קולו ~ 1
ויחדד תנועתיו שעה אחר כך ישפיל ־
המנגן קולו על התדרגות ויריפה מיתריו ~
ויניח תנועתיו אחר כך ישקע בשינה ־
ויפסיק שכבר זכרו הרופאים והפילוסופיס 5
שהשינה על זה הדרך עד שיחיו תנועות
המיתריס הן שמי שנן מקנים לנפש טבע
טוב ומרחיבין אותה מאד ויתיפר בזו ~
ההנהגה לגוף ובשיעור יתעסק אחר זה
שאריתיומן כמה שירתה מקריאה או 10
סיפור עם מי שאוהב לשבת עמו וזהן היות
טוב וכל וישיבתמי שאוהב ישיבתן עמו
לחשיכותן או להתשרן בראייתן או לקלות
דעתן שכל זה מרחיב הנפש ומרחיק ~
ממנה רוע המחשבה ואם היה המנהג 15
עתן בלקיחת מזון אחר בערב יוקח שיעור
חמשים דרהס מהיין וסוכר מזוג כי דרהס

12: ורל]‏ ‏.וכשיעור Should read וכשיעור.‏ 9: ובשיעור]‏ Should read ויתיפה.‏ 8: ויתיפר]‏ .התדרגות :3
Abbreviation of الموصوف‎.‏ Erroneous translation of‏ .רוצה לומר וסוכר‏ 17: ולסוכר]‏

132

1 for sleep, and the chanter should intone with the strings and raise his voice
and continue his melodies for an hour. Then, the chanter should lower his
voice gradually, loosen his strings and soften his melody until he sleeps
5 deeply, whereupon he should stop. Physicians and philosophers have
already mentioned that sleep in this manner, when the melody of the
strings induces sleep, endows the psyche with good nature and dilates it
greatly, thereby improving its management of the body. Upon awakening,
10 he may be engaged for the rest of his day in reading whatever he wishes, or
be attended by someone whose company he chooses. The best is the attend-
ance of someone whose company is desirable because of his virtues, or the
delight in beholding him, or his lightheartedness. All these dilate the psyche
15 and remove evil thoughts from it.

If it is customary by habit to partake of another meal for supper, there
should be taken a measure of fifty drams of the drink described, mixed with
ten drams

---

  1   sleep: The word "sleep," as noun or verb, occurs in the treatise seventeen
times. Here, as in the *Regimen*, the therapeutic use of music is stressed by the
author. See Farmer, 1933.

2 and 4 melodies: In Hebrew, "movements," in this case meaning "melodies."

  4   sleeps deeply: Here Maimonides contradicts his own prescription, "one
should not sleep during the day," as given in his Code, *Mishneh Torah, Hilkot
de'ot*, IV, 5. See the Mishnaic admonition in *Ethics of the Fathers*, III, 10.

  5   Physicians and philosophers: The author is almost certainly referring to the
ideas of Pythagoras and his school. See *Iamblichus*, 1818, Chap. XV, pp.
31–33, where a description very similar to our text is given of the effects of
music on the soul and on sleep, both in the evening and the morning.

  11   whose company he chooses: Advice based on psychological insight.

13–14 lightheartedness: To put the patient in a good humor.

  17   the drink: The Hebrew text incorrectly gives the word for "sugar" (וסוכר),
instead of the word for "described" (כנזכר), possibly because the characters
are somewhat similar.

מי ורד וכ דרהם שׁרש לשון שׁורﬞ﬩וייקח
מעט אחר מעט עד שיגע עת מאכל הערב
וימתין שיעור וצי שעהﬞ עד שיצא היין ﬩
מהﬞ צטומכﬞ ויאכל כמנהגן א﬩ מהתבשלין
הנזכרים אחר כך יבא המנגן כנגונים
שתי שעות אחר המאכל ויסב ויﬠנﬠה
המנגן שירחק מתﬧין ועשמין אחר כך
יישן וישקﬞﬞ ויפסיק מר כמן שעשה
ביומס ואם לא היה המנהג שיאכל בערב
ולא יקח מזון בﬡחר מה שלקח ביומס
ימזוג היין ﬠל היחם הקורﬞ ולﬡ יסור
﬩הלﬡקח ממנו מעט אחר מעט והיתﬧיים
יעשן כעשﬦיהﬦ עד שתגﬠ השינה אﬦ
אחר שתי שעﬦות מהלילה ﬡו גﬞ ﬡו דﬞ דּ﬩
מה שﬠﬧﬦן לו הישיבה ואל יחוש לשיﬠﬧ
מה שיﬦﬦﬡן מהﬦﬠﬦﬦ המזוג כמן שﬠﬦﬦר
כשלﬡﬦﬠﬦ וﬡדּ﬩ﬠ לﬦקﬦ ממנו לﬞ דﬧדּ﬩ﬦ﬙ אדּ

8: וישקט .   12: מהלקח] The word הלוקח has been corrected by a later hand to מהלקח.   13: אם]
Canceled by a later hand.   17: די] According to the Arabic text, should read בﬞ.

1 of rose water and twenty drams of water of oxtongue; this should be taken
little by little until suppertime draws near. He should wait for half an hour
until the drink leaves the stomach, and sup as is his custom on one of the
5 dishes mentioned. Then the chanter should attend and distract him with
songs for two hours after the meal; he should recline and command the
chanter to soften his string and his melodies until he sinks into sleep. The
melody should be stopped as it was done in the daytime.
10 If there is no supper, and if he does not take a second meal after that
taken during the day, he should mix the drink according to the preceding
proportions. He should continue taking it little by little while the strings
play, until sleep draws near, either after two hours of the night, or three or
15 four, as he pleases. If he does not take supper, there is no need to pay
attention to the amount that he takes of the mixed drink. Even if he takes
two

1 oxtongue: The Hebrew translator here adds the word "root" in accordance
with the then prevailing opinion that the root contained the active principle.

3 half an hour: The short interval is explained by the speed of absorption of
alcohol from the stomach.

5 and distract him: Missing in the Hebrew text.

15 no need to pay attention to the amount: The rationale as given in the Hebrew
version (see first note to line 17) is more acceptable: an increase in the amount
of the electuary would encourage sleep.

17 if he does not take supper: This phrase is replaced in the Hebrew translation by the words "If he does not sleep," As this change is also found in
the Latin version, the assumption that the latter was taken from the Hebrew
is further strengthened (see our introduction, p. 11).
two or three hundred: The Hebrew scribe incorrectly gives the number four
instead of two.

135

או ג׳ מאות דרהם או יותר מזה מעט ~ 1
בלילי ימות הגשמים שזה טוב ומרטיב
לגוף ואם היה המנהג שלא יקח שום דבר
עליהין לא יפתיר במעש גרעיני פסתק ″
קלוי כמי לומי או מלח מעט קליפת ~ 5
אתרוג מרוקח בסוכר או כסברתא קלויה ·
הוא הנכון ואם היה המנהג בלקיחת מעט
מהמאכל על היין יותר טובמה שיקחהו ″
תרגולין צלויס בשטר ויהין אותם התרנגולין
אבוסיס כמו שזכרנו בקמח שעוריס ~ 10
וחלב ותאנס וגרעינ החטיס ואל יחשב
מחשב שההפטריה בקליפת האתרוג ~
המרוקח בסוכר מחמם המזג שקליפת
האתרוג שוה בין החוס ובין הקור והיא
רפואה לבית יסמך להפטיר בה וכשיהיה 15
מהבקר השיעור מהשינה יגהיג זו ″
ההנהגה עצמה ולא ישנה שום דבר

1 or three hundred drams of it, or a little more than that on winter nights, it will be good and moistening to the body. It would be best if he made it a
5 habit to eat nothing with the drink, except some kernels of pistachio roasted in lemon juice or salt, or in a citron peel preserved in sugar, or with roasted kernels of myrtle or roasted coriander.

If it is customary to partake of some food after the drink, then it is best to take young chicken broiled on a spit. These should be those young
10 chickens that were fed, as we have mentioned, with barley flour, milk, figs and grains of wheat.

Let no one suppose that taking citron peel preserved in sugar heats the temperament, because the peel of the citron is intermediate between the
15 hot and the cold; it is a cardiac medicament, and he should rely upon taking it.

If he were to start this very regimen as of tomorrow, upon awakening from sleep, he should not alter it in any way

4   except: The Hebrew version substitutes "but will end with" (*yaftīr*). Indeed, pistachio kernels and similar nuts help to neutralize gastric acidity after a drink.

6   roasted kernels of myrtle: This is omitted in the Hebrew text.

10   as we have mentioned: A summary of his instructions on 149*v*.

15   cardiac medicament: Antisyncopal drugs used in the Middle Ages possessed a strong odor.

taking it: Again the Hebrew version substitutes "ending with it" (the meal).

17   any way: Following this, some two pages between 154*v* and 155*r* are missing in the Hebrew text.

Here the Hebrew text is missing.

The numbers of the lines in the running commentary refer to the English version.

1 during the cold season.

Upon arising from sleep he should examine his condition. If there is thirst, drinking oxymel of roses is preferable to drinking hydromel. If there is a little unripening in the urinal, drinking oxymel of currants is preferable.
5 If there is fullness in the stomach, taking ten drams of preserved roses and four drams of that Itrifal is preferable.

On the day in which he decides upon the bath, he should, at its beginning, take the drink as above, and he should reduce the vigor of the exercise and shorten its duration. He should enter the bath immediately after the
10 exercise, then leave the bath and partake of a brew prepared with pomegranate seeds, sugar, many spices, and a touch of hot spices like clove and mace, or a syrup of roses or sorrel, with water of oxtongue, or the syrup

4 (*of the English translation*)

unripening in the urinal: This expression leads to the very beginnings of metabolic concepts in antiquity and the Middle Ages. The notion of "coction," so often found in Galen, was applied to the normal metabolism of the body; "unripened" or "crude" matter, as observed, for example, in the urine and feces, was interpreted as a sign of disease. Our treatise offers examples of these pathological conditions, by describing the disturbances in the "egress of the two superfluities," which thus leave the body in an unassimilated state. "Crude discharges" in bilious disease are mentioned by Hippocrates (*Aphorisms*, VII, 69). The diagnosis of urinary disease was aided by observation of the urinary sediments (*Aphorisms*, VII, 31–35); the bubbles mentioned in Aphorism 34 were possibly later interpreted as albumen in the urine. See also Avicenna, *Canon*, Book 5 (Gruner translation, 1930, p. 326, paragraph 610), where the author speaks of "digestion" (= coction) as a good sign, and "unripening" or absence of digestion signifies disease. The latter state is also designated as crudeness; the Arabic *fadjādja* in our treatise is translated by Dozy, (1881): "crudité (des humeurs)." See also p. 334 in Gruner (1930) and p. 351 on "maturation" with regard to urine, which deals with the "unripening" mentioned in our text.

7 the bath: Hippocrates mentions its "concocting" effect (see next note on "coction") in his *Regimen in Acute Diseases*, LXVI; (vol. II, p. 123 in the Loeb Classical Library edition). Here he uses the words: "It concocts and brings up sputum."

Here the Hebrew text is missing.

The numbers of the lines in the running commentary refer to the English version.

1 which we have compounded and mentioned in the third chapter of that treatise. He should sleep following the bath. Galen said: In ripening what needs be ripened, or in resolving that which is to be resolved, I deem nothing better than sleep following the bath. Upon awakening, he may take food
5 and engage the rest of his day and an hour of the night in what we have mentioned. When the food begins to leave the stomach, he should begin to take that mixed drink, little by little, while the chanter chants, until he sinks to sleep in the manner described. There should be no supper at all that night. If it is customary to have supper, breakfast should be postponed
10 until after arising from the sleep that follows the bath.

As for the time which is selected for coitus, there are two periods

---

2 ripening: Usually rendered as "coction" or "maturation," is mentioned very often by Galen, for example, in *De methodo medendi*, Book XII, (K. X: 823–824), where the salutary influence of sleep which "helps to complete the digestion of the crude humors" is described. The "ripening" and "resolving" refer to biological processes, which were later understood to be metabolic changes.

The rest of this page is more or less a summary of the advice given earlier in the treatise.

אם כשיתאכל המאכל אחר לקיחת או

השיעור המוענ מהיין קודם אכילת

הערב או בסון הלילה זה הכלל לא יהיה

זה הפועל בלקיחת לא על רעבון ופניות

האצטומכא ולא על התמלאות האצטומכא

כמאכל וכמוכן שתייתהיין לא ישתה

והמאכל באצטומכא לא נתעכל מפני שהוא

מפנג ויוצאו קודם התבשלן ולא האצטומכא

פנייך צריכה ללקיחת המזון שהוא אז

מחמם המזג וחמס ויכאיב הראש ושורף

הלחות לא כשיתחיל המאכל בעיכול

ובכל שבועיקח מאותה המרקחת

השוה העשייה כאודם ולא יטייל אותו

היום או כיאותן האטריפלא או מאחד

הנסחאות הנזכרת בקאנון מרפאות

המור ואין דרך ללקיחת מרקחת שהיה

בה שעס דבר כהג עד באדיסתד בשום

1
5
10
15

1: או] Should read אותו (part of the page damaged).   4: בלקיחת] Deleted by a later hand.
8: מפנגו] Should read מפגנו.   9: פנייה.

1 either following digestion of the food after taking the small measure of the drink before supper, or late at night. The crux of the matter is that this action
5 should take place neither during hunger upon an empty stomach, nor when the stomach is filled with food. It is the same with respect to the drink; it should not be drunk before the food in the stomach has been digested, because it will unripen it and expel it before its ripening, or while the stom-
10 ach is empty and in need of food, since at that time it will heat the temperament, cause headache, and inflame the humors. Rather it should be taken when the food begins its digestion.

On each Friday morning, he should take one miskal of that temperate
15 electuary which is prepared with jacinth or of Iṭrīfal, or of one of the recipes of the musk medicaments mentioned in the Canon. He should not exercise on that day. He ought not, by any means, to take an electuary in which there is any castoreum,

1   digestion of the food: The beginning of the passage is not found in the Hebrew text, because it appeared on the missing page, after 154v. The phrase following it deals with the times when intercourse should take place.

3   The crux of the matter: In Hebrew: "This is the rule."

8   unripen: The food is not yet ripe, not sufficiently digested. When a drink is taken before the food in the stomach has been digested, the food remains "unripe," that is, hard (see Kroner's translation, 1928, "verhärten").

9–10   while the stomach is empty: In this case the gastric mucosa absorbs the alcohol in the drink too readily.

10   inflame the humors: This process is described in the old humoral terminology.

12   each Friday: In Hebrew: "each week."

13–14   not exercise: Following the weekly dose of the medicine, the patient should rest, possibly because of the tranquilizing and slightly narcotic effects of the medicament.

143

פעם לאיסיר הגרבאסתר מכל רפואה של 1
מור שיקח ממנו אדוננו זו הנהגת הדמך ~
שיהיה האויר בו קר אבל בזמן החום אליעזר
מהשיעה כי אם אחר שעה מהיומם ויקח
אבתמסא-ה כהמשקים הסכנגבין של ורד 5
והעמוקי והמשקה שזכרעהן בפ.הג מאות
המאמר ויעייל בקר האויר וידון כתבשילם
העשיס אל הקור ויישן דלן אורך מתוך
שמי נגתהיתריס כמו שקדם ולאיקח אית
היין המזוג אם מעט ולא ישכיס בלילה 10
וימעט   המשגל מהרגל החורף ונקדת
רפאות המור הקר שזכרעה חלא מליקחת
רפואת האודם השוה ואם רעה לשטות
שוס דבר מהדין יהיה בסוף הימים
עד שיקח ממנו השיעור הנזכר ויישן 15
נתחלת הלילה או בסוף השעה השטת
ממנו ואם לקח מרפאות האודס הקר

1: הגעדבאסתד] Should read הנעדבאדסתר.   6: בפ] Abbreviation for בפרק   11: וימעט] After this, the next word is corrupted.

1 and castoreum should be omitted from any musk medicament that our Master takes.

This is the regimen for the cold season.

In the hot season, he should not be awakened from sleep except after an 5 hour of the day, and he should take the syrups of oxymel of roses and currants, and the syrup we have mentioned in the third tract of that treatise. He should exercise in the coolness of the air, and breakfast on dishes inclining toward coldness. He should sleep long from listening to the strings 10 as mentioned before. He should take but very little of that mixed drink. He should not pass the night awake and he should reduce coitus below what is customary in the winter. He should take the cool musk medicament we have mentioned instead of the temperate jacinth medicament. If he desires to drink one of the drinks, let it be the end of the day, so that he will take 15 the stated measure of it, and sleep at the beginning of the night or at the end of its second hour. It is good for him to take the cool jacinth medicament.

3 Here begins the regimen for the hot season.

4 after an hour of the day: Because the sun rises early.

8 sleep long: Because of the longer days.

10 but very little: In summer the intake of a drink containing ingredients thought to exert a strong pharmacological action should be reduced. A similar precept has already been expressed on 145*v*, 14.

the night awake: He should not rise too early (according to the Hebrew version).

15 sleep at the beginning of the night: Again the musk or jacinth medicaments should be taken late in the day, because of their hypnotic effects.

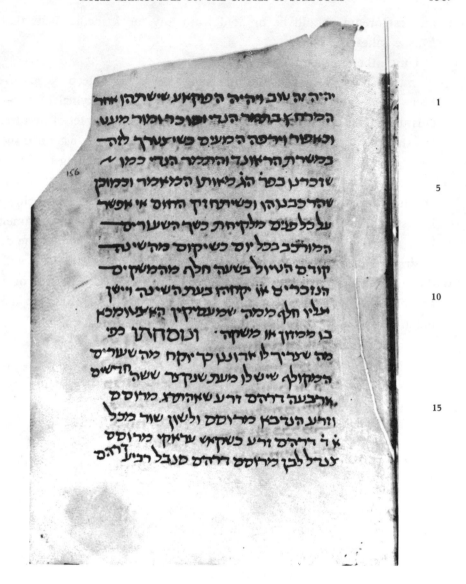

5: בפֿר] Abbreviation for בפרק.   וכמוכן] Following this, the equivalent for الشراب is missing.   15: ארבעה] Should be ארבעים.   17: אֹ] Abbreviation of ארבעה אחד.   כשקאש] Should be spelled כשכאש خشخاش.   מרוסס] Following this, درهمين شني דרהם is missing.

1   The brew that he drinks after the bath should be of tamarind, sugar, musk, and a little camphor.

Softening of the stools, when needed, should be with the infusion of 5 rhubarb and tamarind we have mentioned in the third chapter of that treatise, or with the syrup we have compounded.

If the heat increases, there is no escape from taking barley *kashk*, prepared every day. Take it upon arising from sleep, an hour before the exer-10 cise, instead of the drinks mentioned, or take it at bedtime and sleep upon it, instead of foods or drinks that fill the stomach. Its description in accordance with the needs of our Master is as follows: Take polished barley, six 15 months after it is harvested, forty drams; chopped seeds of fumitory, chopped seeds of endive and oxtongue, of each four drams; chopped seeds of Iraqi poppy, two drams; chopped moistened white sandalwood, one dram; nard, a fourth of a dram;

1   The brew: After the warm bath a special drink is prescribed. This is also meant to restore water-balance after excessive sweating.

5   of that treatise: Refers to the *Regimen*.

7   barley: The time-honored recipe, so often used by Hippocrates.
    kashk: In the Latin translation of the *Canon:* "Kist hordei."

11 that fill the stomach: Overfilling of the stomach is frequently censured by the author (*Hilkot de'ot*, 4:15; *Treatise on Asthma*, Chapter 6).

15 forty: Rendered incorrectly in Hebrew as four.

    chopped: Translated by Kroner "gestossen" (pounded in a mortar).

17 seeds of Iraqi poppy: These perhaps contain a small amount of opium.

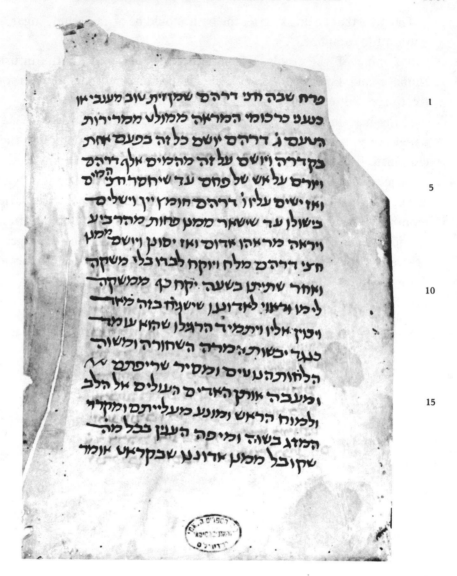

1: שבה] Should be spelled שבת שיִت .مغربي מענבי] Should be spelled מערבי مغربى .4: על זה]
Following this, the equivalent of القدر is missing. 18: שבקראט] This spelling is in accordance with MS. Poc. 280 (Neubauer 1270⁵) בקראט, while in MS. Uri 555 the name
appears as ابقراط Abukrāt (Hippocrates).

148

1 dill flowers, half a dram; olive oil from the Maghrib or Syria, yellow of
   color and free from bitter taste, three drams. The whole of these should be
5 put together in an earthen pot. Pour into this pot one thousand drams of
   water, and heat it over a charcoal fire until half the water evaporates. Then
   pour into it six drams of wine vinegar. Its cooking is completed when less
10 than a fourth of it remains, and its color appears red. Then filter it, and
   add to the filtrate half a dram of salt. It should be taken, alone without
   a drink, and an hour after it is taken, a spoonful of lemon syrup should be
   taken as an electuary.

   It behooves our Master to be most concerned about this, to adopt it and
   to use it habitually, because it will resist the dryness of the black humor,
15 moderate the inflamed humors, remove their burning, thicken those vapors
   that ascend to the heart and the brain, prevent their ascent, cool the temperament through moderation, and improve the condition in all that of which
   our Master complains. Indeed, Hippocrates says

   [End of Jerusalem MS.]

1 dill:Rendered as "anetum" in the Latin translation. Anetum mixed with
   olive oil is mentioned by Galen (K. XI: 832).
   Maghrib: Misspelled in Hebrew (ma‘anavi instead of ma‘aravi).

5 heat it over: In Hebrew "raised over."

9–10 Following the word "salt", the English translation omits the words: and it
   should be taken alone, without the drink, and an hour later.

15–16 to the heart and the brain: This association is exemplified in the modern
   concept of arteriosclerosis, which may give rise to both coronary and cere-
   bral disease.

18 Hippocrates says: The Hebrew manuscript ends abruptly at this point.

   Hippocrates: As previously mentioned, Hippocrates enlarges on different
   medicinal uses of barley, as in his Regimen in Acute Diseases, Chapters X to
   XXVI. In Littré's edition the word "orge" (barley) occupies three columns of
   the index (X: 714–715), and one column is devoted to bread (p. 719). See our
   medical contents, p. 21.

The last pages of the treatise,
which are missing in the Hebrew text

in summation of his enumeration of the virtues of the barley kashk, that it delivers what ought to be to what must be. Our Master should not neglect recourse to it in the summertime in any wise, unless there is constipation, or acidity in the stomach, or flatus beneath the ribs. Whereupon, at such times, our Master should not take it.

Chapter 22   This Servant realizes that because of the excellence of the intellect of our Master and the soundness of his understanding, he is able to regiment himself as is proper, according to that preceding treatise and these chapters, and all the more so if there is at hand someone of whose knowledge he seeks advice, and of whose familiarity with the Art he asks help.

God the All Highest is the Witness, and He is a sufficient witness, that it was the highest hope of this minor Servant to undertake to serve his Master

---

The phrase referring to the barley preparation, "that it delivers what ought to be to what must be," is ascribed to Hippocrates in our treatise. It presumably indicates that it supplements deficiencies or corrects dyscrasias. One of the Latin translations of our treatise (the Vatican MS.) renders the phrase as follows: "Hippocrates dicit . . . quoniam inducit quaequidem cui debet," which is similar to our own interpretation given above. As a general medical principle, it implies that therapeutic measures ought to be carefully considered according to the symptoms and constitution of the individual patient, a practice which Maimonides strongly advocates throughout the treatise.

The deliberations on medicine and religion at the end of the treatise have been commented on by the Maimonides scholars Kroner (1924) and Meyerhof (1929). The liberal attitude of the author, in leaving to the patient the decision whether or not to follow medical advice, does not correspond with his very authoritative manner

by his body and words, not through his paper and quill, but his poor original temperament and his weak natural build — if when young, how much more so in old age — stood between him and many pleasures. I do not mean pleasures, but good, the greatest and most sublime of which, is to undertake the service of our Master. And God is Praiseworthy in all events, the totality of which occur in the totality of existence, and its particulars in each and every person, in accordance with His Will which follows His Wisdom, the depth of which man can not fathom. Praise be to God, always, in any condition, whatever direction events may take.

Let not our Master censure his minor Servant for what he has mentioned in this his treatise about the use of wine and song, both of which the Law abhors, because this Servant has not commanded that this ought to be done, but mentioned what his Art determines. The lawgivers have already known, as the physicians have known, that wine can be of benefit to mankind. The physician, because he is a physician, must give information on the conduct of a beneficial regimen, be it unlawful or permissible, and the

---

as expressed in his other writings (Leibowitz, 1957). Thus, one of the last paragraphs of his health rules (*Hilkot de'ot*, 4, 20) reads:

> 'Whoever lives in accordance with the directions I have set forth, has my assurance that he will never be sick till he grows old and dies; he will not be in need of a physician, and will enjoy normal health as long as he lives—unless his constitution be congenitally defective, or he has acquired bad habits from his early childhood, or if the world should be visited by pestilence or drought'.

In his belief in the efficacy and health-bringing properties of therapeutics, Maimonides took a firm stand, in contradistinction to Rabbi Judah ha-Levi (?1075–1141), the great Hebrew physician-poet, who was a skeptic and not far removed from the "therapeutic nihilism" of the mid-nineteenth century Vienna School (see his beautiful poem "The Physician"; English translation by Salaman, 1924, reprinted 1946, p. 113; German translation by Geiger, 1851, p. 30, and by Rosenzweig, 1925, p. 73, supplemented by a comment on p. 212).

sick have the option to act or not to act. If the physician refrains from prescribing all that is of benefit, whether it be prohibited or permissible, he deceives, and does not deliver his true counsel. It is manifest that the Law commands whatever is of benefit and prohibits whatever is harmful in the next world, while the physician gives information about what benefits the body and warns against whatever harms it in this world. The difference between the edicts of the Law and the counsels of Medicine is that the Law commands compliance with what benefits in the next world and compels it, and forbids that which harms in the next world and punishes for it, while Medicine recommends what is beneficial and warns against what is harmful, and does not compel this or punish for that, but leaves the matter to the sick in the form of consultation; it is they who have the choice.

The reason for this is manifest. In Medicine, the harm of what is harmful and the benefit of what is beneficial, are tangible, immediate, and require neither compulsion nor punishment, while neither the harm nor the benefit

---

The almost dogmatic belief of Maimonides in therapy led him to recommend wine in this treatise. However, in the closing paragraph he must have been conscious of the possible religious scruples of his patient, which prompted this mitigating and more flexible final section. Both Kroner and Meyerhof consider it an act of diplomacy dictated by the situation. Recently our collaborator in this edition, Klein-Franke, 1970, has suggested that Maimonides was safeguarding the free choice of the patient and respecting his conscience. However, the "doctor's dilemma" should be considered in its historical setting, which was so different from that of our times. Now physicians have changed their attitudes about the intrinsic value and irrevocable indication of a certain remedy or a medical treatment, unless these are demanded in an emergency.

As exemplified by the passage from his health rules quoted above, Maimonides used his power of persuasion to induce patients to follow his medical advice; but he never went so far as to lay down the law, as he did in his religious writings. This

of these commands and prohibitions of the Law can be ascertained in this world. The ignorant might well imagine that all that is said to be harmful will not harm, and whatever is said to be beneficial will not benefit, because he does not see it at hand. Therefore, the Law compels the performance of the good and punishes for the evil that cannot be ascertained, be it good or evil, except in the next world. All this is benevolence toward us, favor bestowed upon us, compassion upon us for our ignorance, and mercy for the weakness of our comprehension.

This is the measure of what the Servant has envisaged to present unto the hand of him who holds his bondage, may God perpetuate his days; the wisdom of our Master is supreme. Now, this is the end.

Praise be only to God; He is sufficient for men and a most excellent Guardian.

---

attitude may explain the somewhat puzzling wording in our treatise, "the sick have the option to act or not to act." Experience must have shown him that most patients are inclined to defer responsibility to the doctor rather than to follow their own decisions. Toward the end of his career Maimonides, the philosophically-minded physician, might even have harbored some doubts as to whether the medical knowledge of his time had advanced to the standard set by himself of "perfection to the possible limit." This goal, so characteristic of his lofty view of the medical profession and of the qualities required in the practice of medicine, is expressed in his *Treatise on Asthma*, in Chapter 13:

> 'Be cognizant of the fact that medicine is a very essential wisdom for man at any time and at any place, not only during illness but even in full health, so that I would say that nobody can entirely detach himself from medicine. This is valid as long as the physician has attained perfection to the possible limit, to him will one deliver one's body and soul to be guided by his advice'.

153

THE EXTANT ARABIC MANUSCRIPTS

M. PLESSNER

FOUR MANUSCRIPTS of the Arabic text are known; one of them is incomplete. Only three manuscripts, all in Oxford, are mentioned by Steinschneider (1902, [§]158, Number 21). He could not have known of the existence of a fourth manuscript in Paris, because Zotenberg's description of this codex (1866, No. 1211) is not complete. Two of these four manuscripts are in Arabic script and the other two, including the incomplete copy, are in Hebrew letters.

In the introduction to their English translations of the *Regimen* and of our treatise, Bar-Sela and his collaborators (1964, p. 15) have designated the Arabic manuscripts they consulted as A1 ff., the Hebrew manuscripts as H1 ff., and the Latin manuscripts as L1 ff. As far as the Arabic manuscripts of our treatise are concerned, they only made use of the two in Arabic script; for those two we have retained the designations A1 and A2, to avoid confusion. As the letter "H" has been used by them to indicate the Hebrew texts, I have designated the Arabic manuscripts in Hebrew script as Par(is) and Neub(auer), respectively. I have, unfortunately, not been in a position to provide a complete critical apparatus for Kroner's Arabic text (1928, pp. 33–54),[1] which is here mechanically reproduced, so that the designations introduced by me will only appear in this essay. I hope to publish a full *apparatus criticus* elsewhere.

I first describe the four Arabic manuscripts one by one, taking into account the work already done on them, and I then try to define their relationship to one another. Finally, I provide a few examples of suggested corrections to Kroner's text and to the English translation. Kroner's German translation (1928, pp. 62–85) needs to be completely revised, because its textual basis was too restricted.

THE MANUSCRIPTS

1. A1 = MS. Bodl. Pocock[2] 313, Cat. Uri 555, (*Bibl. Bodl.*, 1787), used in microfilm. At the end of the main text, fol. 53, is the colophon of the scribe, Muḥammad b. ʿAlī b. Abi l-Qāsim b. Khalīl of Damietta, with the date 10. (?) Muḥarram 741 = 6.

---

[1] See Meyerhof's criticism in *Der Morgen*, 1928, 4: 620–622 and his analysis of the work in *Essays on Maimonides*, New York, 1942, pp. 283–285. Baruch in *Janus*, 1969, 56: 257 f., does not even describe the contents of the work correctly.

[2] This is the correct form of the name and not "Pococke"; cf. C. A. Nallino, *RSO*, 1925, 10, 438 n.1 (= *Raccolta di scritti*, 1948, 6, p. 224 n.1). The staff of the Bodleian Library still give the incorrect spelling.

(?) July 1340. The complete text of the colophon, insofar as it is legible, is to be found on pp. 25 f. of Kroner's edition, where it was edited and translated with the help of Enno Littmann. On fol. 3r, which is the first page written in the hand of the main text (the manuscript contained a number of empty pages, which were later filled with prescriptions and the like by other hands), there is the following report by the scribe of his commission to produce this copy.

أُمِرَ بِإِنْشَاءِ هَذَا الْكِتَابِ الْمُبَارَكِ الْمَيْمُونِ إِنْ شَاءَ اللّٰهُ تَعَالَى

الْعَبْدُ الْفَقِيرُ إِلَى اللّٰهِ ﷻ وَجَلَّ الْجَنَابُ

الْكَرِيمُ الْعَالِي الْمَوْلَوِيُّ الْأَمِيرِيُّ الْأَجَلُّ الْكَبِيرُ

الْمَخْدُومِيُّ الْعَا... بْنُ وَلَدِ جَنَابِ الْمَرْحُومِ

الْعَالِي الْأَمِيرِيِّ لِأَجْلِي الْعَزِيزِ مُحَمَّدِ ... الَّذِي أَيَّ نِعْمَاهُ

اللّٰهُ بِرَحْمَتِهِ، وَأَسْكَنَهُ فَسِيحَ جَنَّتِهِ، وَغَفَرَ لَهُ وَلِوَالِدَيْهِ

وَلِجَمِيعِ الْمُسْلِمِينَ وَصَلَاتُهُ ...
وَالِدِهِ وَعَمِّهِ ...
وَحَسْبُنَا اللّٰهُ وَنِعْمَ الْوَكِيلُ

The terms *al-janāb al-'ālī* and *al-amīrī* are documented by Björkman (1928, pp. 126 and 112). According to the latter reference, it appears that another form, *al-ajallī*, is not unprecedented. On the other hand, it was impossible to trace the name of the (father of the ?) person who commissioned the copy. Neither it nor the *nisba* exist; the latter may be *al-Kurānī*, although this name does not fit geographically and is, moreover, graphically unlikely.

In the margin of the first line of this preamble, we read the following words, obviously written by another hand: *al-ḥamdu lillāhi*, "Praise be to God!" and below this, three times, *yā kabīkaj*. This last invocation is frequently to be found on title-pages, as has recently been remarked by Dietrich (1966, p. 41 n.). Of the various meanings of the word given by Steingass (1892), some of which appear to be incompatible with each other, Dietrich singles out "King of the cockroaches" as the most likely. However, he passes over what we consider to be a far more plausible meaning provided by Steingass: "the patron angel of reptiles," which is a poor rendering of the explanation found in Vullers (1855–1867): *nomen genii s. angeli,* *qui reptilibus praeest* (نام ملكى است موكل بر حشران). The term "reptiles" obviously denotes creeping things in general, including bookworms, which are to be banned by the demon. For evidence of the correctness of this interpretation I have to thank Mr. E. Wust, of the Jewish National and University Library, who has shown me the formula *yā kabīkaj iḥfaz al-waraq*, that is, "O Kabīkaj, protect the paper!" on an anonymous and so far unidentified commentary to al-Fargānī's poem *Bad' al-amālī* (Brockelmann, 1937–1942, I: 764) from the A.S. Yahuda Manuscript Collection in the Library.

Kroner's description of the two Maimonides texts in the codex used by him need not be repeated here, but it should be noted that in the *Fī tadbīr aṣ-ṣiḥḥat*, p. 102 (p. 2 of the offprint), the Uri number quoted as 505 should read 555.

2. A2 = MS. Bodl. Huntington 427, Cat. Uri 608. We possess a microfilm of the complete codex, as well as a white on black photograph of the text dealt with here (80v–91v). Fol. (i)r contains only the following, written in Steinschneider's handwriting: *Urii Moh(amedanus) DCVIII. Hunt. 427.* The subsequent leaves up to (vii)r are empty. On (vii)v is written only: *Comm. in Hippocr. auctore Maimonide ut ex collatione cum versione hebr. primus detexi (Steinschneider).* On fol. 1r the *Commentary on the Aphorisms of Hippocrates* by Maimonides starts; the beginning of which is missing. Above it is written in Latin: 10. *Robertus Huntingdon* [*sic*]. Still further up is a table of contents of the whole codex, in an oriental hand differing from that of the scribe of the manuscript. As far as I know, this is now reproduced for the first time:

فهرست : شرح فصول ابوزراط ، مقالة موسى ابن (عبة) عبيد الله الاسرائيلي
القرطبي في البواسير ، وله في الجماع ، وله مقالة في حبس الطبيعة ، وله
رسالة في بيان بعض الاعراض وجوابها ، وله مقالة في ما يبادر به المسوع
من التدبير

The first of these six treatises (Steinschneider, 1902, [§] 158, Number 19), which is the only one to be still unedited, continues until fol. 51r. I noted in *Kirjath Sepher,*

1963, 38: 302, note*, that a portion of the text is missing here. However, the gap between fol. 17 and 18 was not mentioned there, because I was under the impression that this missing piece had later been written in the margin of fol. 17v. As I then possessed a microfilm copy only of the *Commentary on the Aphorisms* and not of the entire codex, I could not know that this addendum came from a different commentary on the *Aphorisms*. I have now found a part of this latter text at the end of the codex (see below). Thus, following fol. 17 there is a gap which someone has perhaps attempted to fill with a piece from another commentary.

The second work begins on fol. 51v (Steinschneider, 1902, Number 14). It has been edited and published by Kroner as "Die Haemorrhoiden in der Medizin des XII und XIII Jahrhunderts," (1914). It breaks off on fol. 54v of this manuscript with the words وقد الفت لسيدنا (Kroner, p. 650, or p. 6 of the offprint, line 18). Folios 55–60 are empty. On fol. 61 is the end of the third work (Steinschneider, 1902, Number 15; edited by Kroner in *Janus*, 1916, 21: 203 ff., and compare O. Rescher's textual corrections in *MSOS*, 1918, 21: 129–131). The fourth work headed *Maqāla fī ḥabs aṭ-ṭabī'a* in both the table of contents and the text, is *fī tadbīr aṣ-ṣiḥḥa* (Steinschneider, 1902, No. 20). This ends on fol. 80r. It has been edited by Kroner (1923–1925) and has been translated into English by Bar-Sela *et al.* (1964), together with the treatise with which we are dealing here. This last, which is the fifth work of the collection (Steinschneider, 1902, Number 21), starts on fol. 80v and ends on 91v. It has likewise been edited by Kroner (1928). At the end of the text is an undated colophon with the name of the scribe and the same assurance that follows other texts of this codex, to the effect that the work has been collated and copied from the author's original script. Fol. 92r contains only the heading of the sixth and last work given in the table of contents: *Maqāla ṣagīrat al-ḥajm fī mā yubādir bihi l-malsū' min aṭ-tadbīr*, that is, the *Treatise on Antidotes* (Steinschneider, 1902, Number 16), which has been translated and published by Steinschneider under the title, "Gifte und ihre Heilung" (Steinschneider, 1873). The text extends from 92v to 106v.

On fol. 108v, a work in Persian *ductus* starts. This is a *risālat al-mujarrabāt*, that is, a collection of approved prescriptions, by an otherwise unknown Dāwūd al-hakīm. It ends on fol. 114r. On fol. 119v, after a number of empty pages, a treatise on the pulse begins, in a Magrebi hand. The author is Muḥammad b. Aḥmad b. al-'Āṣ al-Andalusī, who is probably the same as the author mentioned by Brockelmann (1937–1942, II: 1029, Number 26), where the name is given somewhat differently. This version of the name only appears in MS. Paris 2038, 2 (title, according to Vajda, 1953, p. 461: *Ma'rifat dalā'il an-nabḍ*). This ends on fol. 131v.

Apparently the codex formerly ended here, because fol. 132v is upside down and bears the stamp of the Bodleian Library and the number 427. The binder seems to have been careless when binding in the extra work which now follows. This section, which starts on fol. 133r, opens with *qāla Abuqrāṭ* and is a fragment of a commentary on the *Aphorisms*, in which the explanations of the author are prefaced by the words *qāla l-mufassir*, just as in the corresponding commentary by Maimonides. As a result, the piece was thought to have been part of a text by Maimonides, with which it was later bound together. From it comes the fragment mentioned above, with which the gap in the margin of fol. 17*v* was erroneously filled. A comparison with Muntner's edition of the Hebrew translation (1961) shows that it must have come from another commentary. The text starts with Aph. II, 43 and ends on fol. 134*v* with the heading, Book 3. The author has not been identified.

3. Par = Paris, Bibl. Nat., Anc. f. 411, Cat. Zotenberg 1211. The catalogue refers to only a single work — the *Treatise on Asthma* — in this collection of treatises by Maimonides. However, Steinschneider has noted that it also contains the *Treatise on Poisons* and the *Regimen sanitatis*. Reuben Levy has dealt with the codex in his paper, "The 'Tractatus de Causis et Indiciis Morborum,' كتاب الاسباب والعلامات attributed to Maimonides" (*Studies in the History and Method of Science*, edited by Charles Singer, 1917, pp. 225–234), Levy reproduces the beginning of the manuscript, Bodl. Marsh 379, Cat. Uri 594. Then he attempts to confirm Steinschneider's assertion that such a treatise by Maimonides does not exist (see Steinschneider, 1893, p. 773). In the old Paris Catalogue our manuscript is entitled *de morborum causis et illorum curatione*, but this was apparently intended only as a general heading for the whole collection, without detailed indication of the works of which it consists. As a result, however, a number of scholars have taken this to be a second copy of a work, presumed to be by Maimonides, which is found in Cod. Marsh 379. Levy claimed to have submitted the quite haphazardly bound Paris manuscript to a "careful examination" and to have found that it contains no less than four works — that is, one more than Steinschneider had attributed to it. Levy also discovered our treatise in the codex, but did not observe the presence of at least two additional works, making at least six in all. Professor G. Vajda has been kind enough to send me a photocopy of his own careful analysis of the codex, which is based upon an examination by Dr. Ernest Mainz. According to this, the treatise contains, apart from the works cited by Levy, the *Treatise on Hemorrhoids* and that on *Coitus*, as well as five folios of which the contents have not been identified.

My former pupil, Dr. Simha Zabari, has since been good enough to check Vajda's analysis of our text by comparing it page by page with Kroner's edition, and she has thereby completely confirmed Vajda's statement. I have received a photograph of this text.[3] It begins on fol. 49*v*, jumps from 50*v* to 100*r* and from 100*v* to 103*r*, and then continues uninterruptedly, ending on fol. 122*v*. At the end of this text is the Arabic original of the prescription for a cough medicine, which Kroner has edited

---

[3] My photograph does not show at the head of the text the erroneous title, תשובות רפואיות which, as confirmed by Professor Vajda on inquiry, was later added by Muntner. The latter published a photograph of this page in his German translation (1966), facing page 32, showing that title which the reader might think belongs to the original text.

and published on page 59 in a Hebrew translation taken from Cod. Berol. Or. Qu. 836 and on page 86 in a German translation.

We have learned through Levy's work about the incorrect title of the manuscript. Vajda only notes: *faux titre et faux colophon.* According to his description, two or three hands are represented in the codex and the *Treatise on Poisons* starts on fol. 123*v* in the hand of the scribe of our treatise. We are therefore unable to say anything about the scribe, or the provenance or dating of the copy, although this information is probably to be found at the end of that treatise. The text is written in an easily legible, oriental hand. The Hebrew letters enable us to determine, in each case how the scribe understood the text. This is not always possible in the case of MSS. A1 and A2, where the diacritical points are often lacking or, if present, are at least doubtful if not obviously incorrect.

4.   Neub = MS. Bodl. Pocock 280, Cat. Uri 78, Neubauer 1270, 5 (Neubauer, 1886–1906). What has just been said about the Paris manuscript also holds true regarding MS. Neubauer. Kroner, who used this text, refers readers to the description of the manuscript given in his edition of the *Treatise on Hemorrhoids* (see above). However, he seems then to have been in the same position as when working on our treatise; being only in possession of that part of the codex with which he was dealing, without ever having seen the rest of the volume. In both cases his comments, although fairly extensive, are thus limited to the character of the script and to the language used. Because I have had at my disposal a microfilm of the entire codex, from the Institute of Microfilmed Hebrew Manuscripts of the Jewish National and University Library, I am able to provide the first systematic description of the codex as a whole.

The present contents of the codex have been briefly but sufficiently indicated by Neubauer. Preceding the texts are a number of unfoliated leaves. On the *recto* of the first and second leaves is written: *Poc. 280 Uri Hebr. LXXVIII.* On the second leaf, below this, is the following table of contents, which appears to refer to an earlier composition of the codex. The poor condition of this leaf, which was stuck on to the manuscript, renders the reading of certain details uncertain:

1   Avi [cennae ?] Poema Arabice
2   Diet & Pathology Arabic
3   Consultation[es] morborum ad Maimonidem Araborum Doctorem
4   Maimonides De Resurrectione mortuorum Hebr.
5   Capitula Abi Nasr Al-Pharabi
6   Libr. de medicamentis . . . Moshe ben Maimon Israelita Cordubensis

Numbers 1 and 2 of this table — the mixture of Latin and English is noteworthy — are no longer to be found in the codex, which still consists of several works (see Neubauer). Number 3 may be our text. Number 4, which is the present Number 1, was not used by Finkel for his edition of *Maimonides' Treatise on Resurrection*,

1939. The present Number 2 is a fragment of the work edited by Steinschneider: מאמר ביחוד (see Steinschneider 1893, [§] 252), which extends here from 13*r* to 16*v*. The new Number 3 (17*r* to 28*v*) is *De coelo et mundo* from Avicenna's encyclopedia, *aš-Šifā* in Hebrew translation (Steinschneider, 1893, [§] 152). The present Number 4 is the *Mikrokosmos* of Josef b. Ṣaddīq ([§] 238, Fragment, 29*r*–32). After a number of empty leaves our text, which is Number 5a of Neubauer's list, begins on fol. 36*r* and ends on 44*r*. In Kroner's edition it starts on page 43, line 18. Number 5b of Neubauer's list (possibly Number 6 of the old table) is the *Treatise on Poisons* of Maimonides in the original Arabic (Steinschneider, 1902, [§] 158, Number 16). It extends from fols. 44*v* to 62*r*. Finally, Number 5c is the text on *Hemorrhoids* (Steinschneider, 1902, [§] 158, Number 14) from fol. 62*v* to 68*r*.

Now follows Number 5 of the old list (Neubauer's Number 6), on fol. 69*r*, headed: הגיון...(?) פרקי אבו נצר אלפראבי (the author's name is throughout spelled thus, without an *alef* following the *pe*) *capitula Abu Nasser alpharabi*. On 69*v* is written: פרקי אבו נצר אלפראבי ז"ל (!). This refers to a Hebrew translation of the Arabic text, *Fuṣūl al madani*, edited by Dunlop in 1961 as *Aphorisms of the Statesman* (see Steinschneider, 1893, [§] 158, Number 3. Here "Uri 178" should read "Uri 78"). At the end of the text, on fol. 91*r*, is a colophon from the year 5223 = 1463. The rest of the contents (Neubauer's Numbers 7 and 8), which are of no interest here, were also not included in the old list.

THE RELATIONSHIP OF THE MANUSCRIPTS TO ONE ANOTHER

The examination of the *variae lectiones* in the four manuscripts shows that manuscript A2 is practically never unique in its *lectio*, but shares it in most cases either with Al or with Par. On the other hand, the reading of Al often differs from that of all the other texts and the same holds good, if less frequently, for Par. Manuscript Neub, which contains only the last three-fifths of our treatise, almost always reads with one or more of the other manuscripts.

Although these results obviate any clear-cut classification of the manuscripts, it must be noted that A1 and A2, the two manuscripts in Arabic script, frequently offer a common *lectio* in which they differ from Par and Neub, which are in Hebrew script, and the latter are, moreover, often joined by the Hebrew translations. On the other hand, in a large number of places A2 reads with the texts in Hebrew script and Par reads with the "Arabic" group. All that can be concluded is that the Hebrew translators seem to have used an Arabic text related to the Arabic manuscripts in Hebrew script.

It follows that it is impossible to rely on any particular "group" of manuscripts when trying to produce as correct and authentic a text as possible. In each case the correct *lectio* must be chosen individually; a task in which the translations are, of course, of great assistance.

Unfortunately, Kroner only had at his disposal A1, the worst manuscript of all.

Due to his command of Arabic and his understanding of the subject-matter of the treatise, he succeeded in correcting most of the text of this manuscript, even including the part not covered by Neub. This is demonstrated in Kroner's *apparatus criticus*, which is here reproduced with his text.

Some examples are given below of what still requires to be done in order to correct the Arabic text and the English translation. These also show that in all probability, the Latin translation was made directly from the Arabic text.

131 A, 14
(Bar-Sela, p. 32, note 2)

All the texts are correct, but the Latin has *regem*, that is, *malik* ("king"), instead of *mālik* ("owner"). This suggests that the translation was taken directly from the Arabic, as Jer. reads *ādōn* — "Lord," which cannot be confused with *melekh*. The Latin has therefore not discarded the place-name Raqqa, as Steinschneider (1893, p. 773) has stated, but has combined the words *mālik* (in this case read *malik*) and *riqqih* into a single expression.

133 A, 13
(Bar-Sela, p. 32b para. 3, lines 4–5)

"advised in this regard" is taken from the incorrect reading in A1 and A2, while Par puts the negation *mā* before the word "advised," which reverses the meaning of the sentence. The correct reading of Par is found in both Jer. and the Latin (*contradicunt*).

134 B, 10
(Bar-Sela, p. 33A para. 2, line 5)

"Andalusia. And all the Arabs . . ." This is taken from the incorrect readings in A1 and A2, *al-'arab* (without a diacritical point), while Par correctly gives *al-gharb*, "the West." Both the Jer. and Berl. Hebrew texts rightly give *ha-'ereb* or *ham-ma'rāb*, "the West." Similarly, the Latin is *in terris hyspanie et in toto occidente*.

148 B, 2–4
(Bar-Sela, pp. 36B– 37A and note 33)

The correction of the text by the translators is based on a misunderstanding. Page 148B, lines 2–4, should be translated: "as the custom goes, *but* (*lākin*) it should [delete the negation] be sifted thoroughly," that is, exactly as given in the rejected version in the note, (see Bar-Sela et al., 1954). This is also the reading provided by Jer. and by the Latin edition of Klein-Franke: *sed excedat in separatione*, and so on. The alteration of the text, on the basis of another work of Maimonides which deals with quite different matters, does not receive the slightest support from any of the texts, all of which are in complete agreement with this interpretation.

(Missing in the Hebrew text. Bar-Sela p. 40B)

In the second half of the page the word "compels" (*yajbur*) is found three times and the word "compulsion" (*jabr*) once. Both Hebrew texts end before this passage, but all the Arabic manuscripts, including those in Hebrew script, contain this meaningless reading. The Law does not "compel"; the sense of the entire passage requires the insertion of the word "recompense," which as *remunerare* appears in all four places in the Latin. It seems that in his copy of the Arabic text the Latin translator found the verb *yajzī* in three places and that in the common source of our Arabic manuscripts this was misread as *yajbur*. In the fourth place, however, the Latin translator must have found *jazā'*, and it is difficult to explain how this word became *jabr* in our Arabic texts. Either the Latin translator or the Arabic scribes must have corrected this word according to their understanding of the verb in the other three places. Be this as it may, the *varia lectio* of the Latin is only possible if it were translated directly from the Arabic and from a manuscript written in Arabic letters.

APPENDIX:

Transmission of the text and Concordance of the Inventory of the Different texts

Ibn Sīnā Mon. 280	Kroner	A1, A2	Par	Neub	Hebr. (H 4)	Jer.	Lat. repr. Freimann, pp. 65–79
	33_{2-15}	+	+	—	55_{2-3}	+	+
	33_{16-21}	+	+	—	55_{5-11}	+	+
	$33_{21}-34_{13}$	+	+	—	55_{12-26}	+	+
	$34_{14}-35_{18}$	+	+	—	56	+	+
	35_{18-19}	+	+	—	57_{7-8}	+	+
	$35_{19}-36_{18}$	+	+	—	—	+	+
	36_{18-19}	+	+	—	57_{10-11}	+	+
	36_{19-22}	+	+	—	—	+	+
	$36_{22}-37_2$	+	+	—	57_{13-14}	+	+
	37_{2-15}	+	+	—	—	+	+
	37_{16-24}	+	+	—	57_{16-25}	+	+
	$37_{25}-38_{11}$	+	+	—	$57_{27}-58_{12}$	+	+
	$38_{12}-39_{20}$	+	+	—	—	+	+
	$39_{21}-40_1$	+	+	—	58_{14-16}	+	+
	40_{2-8}	+	+	—	58_{18-24}	+	+
	40_9-41_{13}	+	+	—	—	+	+	from 40_{17} ed. Klein-Franke
	41_{13-18}	+	+	—	—	+	+
59 pu-61	$41_{18}-43_{19}$	+	+	+	—	+	+
	$43_{19}-46_{19}$	+	+	+	—	+	+
	$46_{20}-47_{16}$	+	+	+	$58_{26}-59_{12}$	+	+
	$47_{16}-49_{19}$	+	+	+	—	+	+
	$49_{19}-50_{19}$	+	+	+	—	—	+
	$50_{19}-52_{17}$	+	+	+	+	+	+
	$52_{17}-54_{10}$	+	+	+	+	—	+
	$54_{15}-54_{22}$	+ ?	+	+	59_{14-20}	—	—

All figures refer to pages and lines of Kroner's edition. (+ = extant, — = not extant).
Occasional missing words have been ignored.

THE ARABIC TEXT

reprinted from the 1928 edition
published by H. Kroner*
(pp 33–54)

* Kroner used the manuscripts Cod. Uri 555 J = Pocock 313
in Arabic letters and Cod. Pocock 280 (Neubauer 1270⁵) in
Hebrew characters, adding some suggestions of variant readings,
given in his text in square brackets.

بسم الله الرحمن الرحيم

ورد على المملوك الاصغر الكتاب المضمن تفصيل تلك الاعراض كلها التى
عرضت لمولانا خلد الله ايامه وتبيين اسباب تلك الاعراض كلها وازمنة/حدوثها
والاخبار بكل جزوية يفتقر الطبيب للسؤال عنها ووصف ما تدبر به فى كل
وقت لكل عرض منها وسطّر فيه ما اشار الاطباء بعمله مما اتفقوا عليه
او اختلفوا فيه.

وعلم المملوك الاصغر علما يقينا ان ذلك الكتاب عن املاء مولانا بلا شك
والمملوك يقسم بالله تعالى ان فضلاء اطباء عصرنا يقصرون عن معرفة ضرورية
نظم تلك الشكية فكيف ان يعبّرون عنها وينظمونها ذلك النظام ولذلك
راى المملوك الاصغر ان يكون جوابه لمالك رقّة ادام الله ظله كلام طبيب
لطبيب لا كلام طبيب لمن ليس هو/من اهل الصناعة.

اذ قد تبيّن للمملوك كمـل مولانا فى معرفة تلك الاعراض واسبابها وقد
علم المملوك تلك الاعراض المستقرة الان وهى التى يرام دفعها وقد ذكره مولانا
للمملوك الاصغر ما اشار به كل طبيب وامره بان يذكر ما عنده فى قول كل
واحد منهم فامتثل ذلك.

1. فصل اما قول من قال من الاطباء لوجاء الدم من افواه العروق الان كما
قـد جاء فى بعض الاوقات لارتفعت تلك الاعراض الموجودة الان فهو قول
صحيح لا ريب فيه وذلك ان ذلك الدم الذى يجىء انما هو عكر الدم وثفله/
والطبيعة تدفعه لرداءته على جهة من جهات البحارين. واما من اشار من
الاطباء بفتح افواه العروق بمياه يجلس فيها او لبائخ يجلس عليها فهو
خطأ ولا يرى المملوك بذلك بوجه لعدّة اوجه بيّنها المملوك اولها لان تلك
الاشياء التى تحمل او تجلس فى مائها حارة فقد ربما اسخنت المزاج وشيطت

131r

131v

132r

167

الاخلاط والثانى ان هـذه العـروق اذا فتحتها الطبيعة فتحتها بتقدير ما Kr 34
يحتاج واذا فتحناها نحن بالادوية فقد تنفتح باكثر مما ينبغى ويفرط سيلان
الدم ويعسر مسكه فقد يعترى ذلك فى الذى يجىء/من تلقاء نفسه وعلى 132v
انه يفرط حتى لا يقدر مسكه والثالث ان هـذه العروق اذا انفتحت من
نفسها فالذى يجىء منها على الاكثر هو الشىء الذى ينبغى خروجه لانه
قـد دفعته الطبيعة (للاقاصى) [للاقاصى] وتحركت القوة الدافعة لدفعه واذا
فتحناها نحن فقد يجىء ما لا ينبغى خروجه وان جاء منه شىء فيكون الذى
يجىء مما لا ينبغى خروجه اكثر وبالجملة فانا لا نلتجىء لهذا الفعل الا اذا
تورمت تلك المواضع وعظم الها جدًّا فنلتجىء حينئذ لفتحها بادوية حتى
يسيل ما اندفع هناك من الدم الذى ورّم تلك المواضع ويكون فعلنا حينئذ
شبيه بفعل من يبطّ ورما لم يمكن الطبيعة ان يفجّر ما على الورم ويخرج ما /133r
فيه ولا ينبغى ان يفعل مولانا هذا بوجه لكنه ان جاء من تلقاء نفسه كما
قد جاء مرات لا يقطع بوجه الا ان افرط وعياذا بالله.

2. فصل ثم ذكر المولى ان بعض الاطباء اشار بتناول شىء من الخمر بماء •
لسان الثور بعد الطعام ساعات وان يتناول منه شىء[a] عنـد النـوم كى
يستغرق فى النوم وان بعضهم اشار بهذا وقال لا وجه لاستعماله اذ الصرف منه
يسخّن المزاج والممزوج يولد الرياح وينفخ. والذى يراه المملوك ان الراى الاول/
هو الصحيح وذلك ان البسير منه وهو اوقيّة شاميّة ونحوها اذا اخذ الطعام 133v
فى الانهضام مما يعين على الهضم ويعين على خروج الفضول بادرار البـول
وينقى عن الدم الابخرة الدخانيّة المولدة لهذه الاعراض الموجودة الان كلها
ولا سيّما اذا مزج بماء لسان الثور واذا انقع فيه لسان الثور نفسه قدر
درهمين فى الاوقيّة كان ابلغ وكان يبسطه النفس اكثر واذا قالت الاطباء
الشراب المفرح باطلاق انما يريد بذلك شراب لسان الثور واذا القى لسان
الثـور فى الشراب زاد فى بسطة النفس/وتفريحه[b] وشرب الخمر يرطب للجسد 134r

_____

a) Besser شفًا.   b) Besser وتفريحها.

Kr 35 رطوبة جيّدة قـد ذكر ذلك جالينوس فى كتابه فى تدبير الصّحّة واما من
زعم انه يسخّن فقد اخطأ لان الخمر غذاء لا دواء وهو غذاء جيّد جدّا
والاغـذيـة الجيّدة لا تسخّن ولا تبرد والادوية هى التى تسخّن وتبرد واما
يتولّد عنه دم محمود على طبيعة الدم الطبيعى الذى هو حارّ رطب واما
مزجه فلا شك انه يولّد ريّاحا وقد ربما ولّد رعشة لكن قد ذكر ابن زهر

134v وهو اوحـد عصره ومن عظماء/المتنعّمين الممزوج يفعل ذلك اذا مزج لحينه
وشرب اما اذا مزج ويترك اثنى عشر ساعة او اكثر وحينيـذ [شرب] فانه
حينئذ جيّد جدّا ان الخمريّة يقوى على الماءيّة ويجيلها ويحسّن المزاج وما
ينصح المملوك هو الذى ينبغى ان يستعمل من لسان الثور وهو قشر اصوله
لا ورقه كما يستعمل اهل الشأم واهل مصر هكذا راينا جميع الشيوخ الفضلاء
يفعلون فى بلاد الاندلس وجميع العرب يصفون قشر اصوله لا ورقه وهذا
النبات ينبغى لمولانا ان لا يفارقه لان له خصوصيّة ببسط النفس ومحو للخلط
السوداوى واستئصال اثره وما جربه المملوك وصحّ صحّة لا شك فيها ان

135r الشراب الرقيق اذا مزج/بيسير ماء ورد قدر العشر فانه يبسط النفس ولا
يسكر ولا يضر بالدماغ ويقوى المعدة ويزيد فى جميع الفضائل المنسوبة الى
الخمر فلذلك يشير المملوك بان يلقى فى (الادوية) [الاوقيّة] الشاميّة من
الخمر عشرة دراهم ماء ورد درهم لسان ثور ويترك عشـر ساعات او
نحوها وحينئذ يتناول واما تناوله ايضا عنـد النوم فنعم الراى لعدّة وجوه
ليستغرق فى النوم ولتذهب الفكر ولحسّن الهصوم وليندفع الفضول.

3. فصل واما اتّفاق الاطّباء على كون المزاج انحرف الى الحرّ وانه ينبغى ان

135v يتناول ما يبرّد ويرطّب فهذا قول صحيح/لكنـه (محمل) [مجمل] ينبغى ان
يفصّل ويذكر التدبير فاما الـذى اشار منهم بشرب الهنـدبا بشراب الصندل
ونقيع التنر هندى واجاص وعناب فيبدو (المملوك) [للمملوك] ان ذلك خطأ
(عظيما) [عظيم] لان هذا التدبير المطلق مع كون البلغم له غلبة فى المزاج
الاصلى لا يليـق بوجه وبخاصّة بالاجاص والعناب فان ذلك يرخى المعدة

169

Kr 36 ويصير بها جدا ويقصّر (الهموم) [الهضوم] واذا رطّبت المعدة وارتخت فسدت

136r الهضوم الثلثة ولا يصلح مثل هذا التدبير الا لمن/غلبت عليه المرة الصفراء
ولم يذكر شيئا يدلّ على غلبة الصفراء بوجه بل المتحصّل من جميع الدلائل
المذكورة هو تولد اخرة سوداويّة حادثة عن سوداء متولّدة عن احتراق بلغم
ينوب بادوار.

٤. فصل واما من اشار بشرب نقيع الراوند فى ماء الهندباء يوم*a* ويترك
يومين فان كان قصد بذلك إلانة الطبع فانه صواب وقد ذكر المملوك صفة

136v تلين الطبيعة/بالراوند فى الفصل الثالث من مقالته التى قد مثلت فى مجلس مولانا.

٥. فصل واما الذى اشار بالاستحمام كل ثلثة من الايام والرياضة فى كل
يوم والتندهن بدهن البنفسج فكل هذا صواب وسينتكلم المملوك فى ذلك
بتفصيل وتقدير.

٦. فصل واما الذى اشار بوضع الخرق المعندئة على الكبد وكذلك من
اشار باكل الخيار والخس والقثّاء والرجلة والاسفاناخ والقطف فكل هذا خطأ

137r محض .وهذا تدبير يصلح لاصحاب الحميات/المحرقة الشديدة التلهب اذا
حدثت بالمحرورى المزاج فى الصيف واشتّ من هذا خطأ من اشار بشرب
اللبن لحليب لانه (لحط) [لحظ] معنى الرطيب ونسى سرعة استحالته لاى
خلط وجد ولم يفكر فى مادة سبب المرض وهو البلغم المحترق.

٧. فصل الذى اشار باستعمال السكنجبين السفرجلى بعد الغذاء بساعة
فهو صواب وتدبير جيد يحسن الهضوم واما اضافته للشراب عصارة برباريس/

137v بعد الطعام فهو تدبير غريب خارج عن مقاييس الطبيّة وعن المعتاد
اعنى تناول عصارة البرباريس والطعام فى المعدة حتى لو كان والمعدة خالية
لا مدخل للعصارة فى هذا المرض.

٨. فصل واما من اشار بشراب المفرح*b* لان (التنلميد) [التنكميد؟] او غيره

---

a) Richtiger يومًا.

b) شراب المفرح wohl einheitlicher Begriff (cf. K. 2): „Freudetrank".

وكذلك من اشار بشراب حماض وتفاح وماء لسان الثور وبزر ريحان وبزر Kr 37

ترنجان فكل هذا صواب. واما اضافته لذلك بزر قطونا فلا يراه/المملوك لانى 138r

لا ارى بتدبير كثير فى هذا المرض وهذا المزاج.

9. فصل واما من اشار بتناول ماء الشعير بخشخاش وبزر يقطين فهو
عجب مع ما ذكره من اعتدال النوم وكان عنده ترطيب ماء الشعير مقصّرًا
حتى رفده ببزر اليقطين واعجب من هذا الذى راى بتناول الاجاص بعد
ماء الشعير ما اظن عند هاولاى الاطباء عضو من اعضاء البدن اخسّ من

المعدة وانه لا يلتفت للمعدة ارتخت/او لم ترتخ حدثت فيها بلة او لم 138v

تحدث او لعلهم يقرّون بشرف المعدة وعموم منفعتها وانه ينبغى ان تصرف
العناية لها دائما ولذلك افرد افاضل الاطباء لها مقالات غير ان هذا التدبير
عندهم يقوى المعدة ويجوّد هضمها ويجفف بلتها ويقطع لزوجة البلغم
الذى لا يبرح يجتمع فيها دائما وهى بينة ويلطف غلظه وهو التدبير تقدّم

ذكره عنهم وهو ماء الشعير ببزر اليقطين والخشخاش وينتقل بعده بالاجاص

واما يسبع/المملوك فى هذا الفصل ما ينبغى تسيعه نبحذر جدّا ولا يحتتّ 139r

لقول قائله جملة.

10. فصل واما تناول التفاح والسفرجل وامتصاص حب الرمان بعد الغذاء
فهذا مأمور به فى حق الناس كلهم عند تدبير الصحّة وليس فى هذا
زيادة تتعلق بهذا المرض الا ما ذكره من تناول كزبرة بعد الطعام فان ذلك
ضحكة بالحقيقة لان قائل هذا قاله لكون الكزبرة تغلظ الابخرة وتمنعها من
الترقّى [الى الدماغ] وذلك حق لكنها ينبغى ان تتناول فى الادوية

كالسفوفات/ونحوها او تطبخ مع الاغذية اما تناول الكزبرة بمفردها بعد الطعام 139v

فان ذلك ان لم يحدث قىء فهو (يغى) [يغثى] بلا شك ويفسد الطعام واما
تناول بزر رجلة بسكر فى بعض الاوقات لا مع الطعام فهو جيد ولو خالط
الطعام ايضا لما ضرّ ذلك فى تبريده وتقويته للقلب.

11. فصل وذكر مولانا ان اشار الاطباء بتناول المشمش واللمثرى والسفرجل

بعد الطعام والعنب والبطيخ والرمان قبله وما علم/المملوك معنى هذه المشورة ‏Kr 38‏ 140r

ان كان القصد انه ان دعت الضرورة للشهوة او العادة لتناول شيء من الفاكهة فينبغى ان يتناول قبل الطعام ما يلين الطبع ويوخذ من الفاكهة بعد الطعام ما فيه قبض كالكمثرى والسفرجل والتفاح فهذا صواب وان كان اشاروا بان تناول هذه الفواكه نافعة لهذا المرض فذلك خطأ لان الفواكه الرطبة كلها رديئة لجميع الاصحاء وللمرضى اذا اخذت على جهة الغذاء وبخاصة البطيخ والمشمش لسرعة استحالتها لاىّ خلط رديء كان فى الجسم وكذلك

/الخوخ رديء جدا وهو مادّة للحميات الرديئة وقد ذكر جالينوس انه منذ 140v قطع اكل الفاكهة الرطبة كلها لم يحم الى اخر عمره وتطول فى حكايته تلك على وجه النصيحة للناس ما هو منصوص فى مقالته تلك فلذلك ينبغى ان يجتنب مولانا الفاكهة الخضراء لجهده.

‏12.‏ فصل الذى اشار باجتناب لحوم الصيد والقديد والباذنجان وكلما يسخن قد اصاب وكل هذه تزيد فى ما شكاه مولانا من الاعراض وكذلك الذى اشار بالرياضة كل يوم وفق جدا ونصح وكذلك الذى نهى عن التوجه للبلاد الحارة نصح فى مشورته واما من زعم ان البلاد/الحارة تحلل ‏141r‏ الابخرة فتلك الابخرة هى التى تترقى لسطح الجسم اذا كانت باردة رطبة واما (هذه) [هذا] الذى يترقى عن دم غليظ عكر فان تلك البلاد تزيد فى غلظ الدم وبسطه وتكثر ابخرته واذا تمكّنت الصحّة ان شاء الله توجه مولانا حيث شاء حتى يكمل الله اماله فى الدارين.

‏13.‏ فصل ولا يرى المملوك الاستفراغ باللازورد ولا بالحجر الارمنى اما اللازورد فلقوّته واما للحجر الارمنى فلكونه مجهول العين وقد شك فيه افاضل الاطبّاء واكثرهم على ان ليس هو هذا الذى يلقب بهذا الاسم وكذلك يستنصوب المملوك رأى من انهى/[a]عن استعمال المسهلات القويّة والاقتصار ‏141v‏ على الراوند او ماء (الجبن) [الجبن] او والسنا مكى ونحوها كل هذا صواب

---

a) Richtiger نهى.

Kr 39 ولا يرى المملوك بنقيع للخوخ ولا بماء البطيخ لاضرارها بالمعدة وليس فيما يشكى

من الاعراض لا تلهب ولا عطش ولا يرى ايضا بالاكثار من النيلوفر لتغليظه

الدم وارخائه المعدة ولا تصلح هذه الا لاصحاب للحميات للحادة الملتهبة كما

142r ذكر المملوك ولا يرى المملوك ايضا باستعمال/مطبوخ الافتيمون لاكرابه وتجفيفه

فان نفع a افتيمون فى مائة (درهما) [درهم] من ماء للجبن وأخذ ذلك مرتين

(ثلات) [او ثلاثا] فى زمان الربيع ومرة فى للخريف او مرتين كان جيدا

ويكون بين كلّ مرة ومرة خمسة عشر يوما ويلبث الافتيمون بدهن لوز

ويصرّ فى خرقة مهلهلة وبعد ذلك ينقع ليلة فى ماء للجبن.

14. فصل وذكر مولانا اذ قد فصد العرق مرة يخرج الدم غليظ[ا] مثل

الطحال فاشار الاطباء من اجل ذلك بالفصد اما بحسب ما يظهر فى وقت

142v دون وقت من الامتلاء/بلا شكّ ان يفصد ويخرج من الدم بحسبه

والذى ينبغى ان (بفصد) [يقصد] دائما هو ترويق الدم وتعديل مزاج

الكبد حتى تتولد دما جيدا وقد بيّن المملوك فى مقالته المتقدمة كيف

يكون ذلك بالاشربة التى ركبها.

15. فصل واما من اشار بكون الاغذية خوخية وتمر هندية بلحوم للجداء

فذلك صواب فى زمان الصيف وينبغى ان لا تغفل لالقاء الدارصينى والمصطكى

والسنبل فى هذه الالوان ونحوها حتى لا تضر بالمعدة وكذلك تناول السلائق

143r المبردة كما اشاروا فى زمان الصيف فان ذلك نحس/بشرط ان لا يكثر

منها ولا يجعل قصد الان b رأى المملوك تعديل المزاج لا الزيادة فى التبريد

اذ والاصل احتراق البلغم.

16. فصل واما من اشار بشراب المفرح ومعجون يكون فيه ياقوت وزمرد

وذهب وفضة فكل هذا صواب ونافع جدا لانها ادوية قلبية تنفع بالخاصية

---

a) Muss wohl نقع gelesen werden: Wenn geweicht wird.

b) Muss wohl verschrieben sein für قصدا لان „und dass es nicht absichtlich
getan wird, weil die Ansicht des Dieners ist".

Kr 40 اعنى بصورتها النوعيّة التى ذلك جملة جوهرعا لا مجرد كيفيتها.

17. فصل واما ما ذكره مولانا من كثرة ما استعمل من ماء لسان الثور والنيلوفر ولم يرتفع بذلك اصل المرض فتعلة فى قلة نفعه كثرة مداومته ولذلك ان الادوية القويّة جدا فى الغاية اذا اديم استعمالها انقلبت الطبيعة ولا يتأثر لها وتصير اغذية او كالاغذية قد ذكر ذلك جالينوس. فتاهيك هـذه الادوية الضعيفة القريبة من (الادوية) [الاغذية] فانها تنولت جمعة

143v متوالية بطلت افعالها الدوائية ولا يظهر لها بعد ذلك /اثره فلذلك ينبغى التنقل من دواء الى دواء واغبب a اندواء نواحد ايلم وحينيذ يرجع له.

18. فصل واما ما ذكره مولانا من تقليل للجماع عن اعتادة فنعم الفعل وما اعظم فائدة هذا التقليل. واما للحمام فلا ينبغى اغبابه بوجه لا فى وقت النوبة ولا وقت الفترات وكون النوم على العادة نعمة كاملة ودليل واضح على كون هـذه الابخرة السوداوية لم تنك الدماغ ولا غيرت مزاجه وانما ينكى فى انقلب خـاصة واما ما ذكره مولانا من وجود الضعف بعـد الرياضة/

144r /فعلة ذلك تركها واغبابها فلو تدرّج فى ارجوع اليها (قليل) [قليلا] بعـد قليل لوجـد عقبها من القوة والنشاط ما يلزم ان يوجـد بعقب كل رياضتة جارية على ما ينبغى.

19. وقد جاوب المملوك الاصغر على جميع ذلك فصول ذلك انكتب انكتيم كما امر فهـو يجمع القول ويؤخّره فى فصل واحد يبيّن فيه كيف يكون تدبير مولانا بحسب هـذه الاعراض الموجودة الان وان كان ذلك تبيّن مما ذكره المملوك فى هـذه الفصول وما ذكره فى تلك المقالة فلنه اقويل متفرقة لا متنسقة وقبل/ان اخذ فى هـذا الفصل اقول انه ينبغى ان يكون فى خزانة

144v مولانا (مضاف) [مضاف] الى تلك الاشربة والاشريفل انتى ذكرها المملوك فى الفصل انثلث من مقلته المتقدمة معاجونين.

a. احدهما دواء مسك بارد قد جرب شيوخ انضب اللذين نثم ذرية فوجد

Kr 41 له فعل عجيب حتى انهم لا يسمعون ببله ووصف لبسائضه بل يدفعون
من عندهم معجونين وهو دواء الفه الرازى فى كتابه فى دفع مضارّ الاغذية.
وهذه صفته بنصّ كلامه يوخذ من الورد المطاحون والطباشير والنزبيرة اليابسة
والكهرباء من كل واحد جزوا ومن اللؤلؤ الصغار نصف جزو ومن المسك الجيد
الخالص سدس جزو يوخذ/من السكر الابيض الطبرزد فيجل بماء التفلح
الحامض المعصور المصفى ويطبخ حتى يصير فى قوام العسل ويطرح فيه اوراق
من اوراق الاترج ويعجن الادوية به ويتعاهد هذا الدواء صاحب هذا
العارض فانه دواء شريف لتقوية القلب من غير اسخان ويعلم للخفقان
واختلاج القلب مع حرارة.

b . والدواء الثانى هو معجون اليقوت التى الفه ابن سينا فى مقالته
المشهورة فى الادوية القلبيّة وذكر منه ثلاث نسخ الواحد بارد والثانى حار
والثالث معتدل والذى يراه الملوك ان الذى يستعمله منها مولانا هو
المعتدل. وهذه صفة الثالث بنصّ كلامه قال تركيب اخر شريف جدا جربته
معجونا واقراصا وزدت ونقصت منه بحسب مزاج مزاج فكان/نفعه فى تقوية
القلب نفعا شديدا وهذه خميرتة نؤؤ كهرباء بسذ من كل واحد درم
ونصف ابريسم مقروص سرطان نهرى محرق من كل واحد مثقال ودانق
نسان انثور خمسة دراهم سحنة الذهب وزن دانقين بزر انفلنجمشل [ك]
بزر البادروج بزر البادرنجوية من كل واحد وزن ثلثة b دراهم بهمن احمر بهمن
ابيض عود هندى حجر ارمنى حجر اللازورد مغسول مصطكى سلجة دار
صينى زعفران عيل بوا قاقلة كبيرة كبةة من كل واحد مثقال افثيمون وزن
درهمين ونصف اسطوخونس c وزن ثلثة دراهم (حدوار) [جدوار] مثقال فان
لم يوجد فبدله d درونج رومى مثقلين بزر الهندباء وزن
خمسة دراهم بزر القثاء وزن اربعة دراهم/مسك مثقلان كافور مثقال عنبر مثقال

---

a) Hier u. ff. für جزء.

Die Laa. des Cod. Pococke 280:   b) Stets תלאתה.   c) אסטכדוס.

d) מתקאלין דרונג.

Kr 42 سنبل سانج هندى من كل واحد رزن درهمين فهذا هو الاصل والخمير فقد

يقرص وقد يجمع بالعسل وكلاها قد يعمل بحسب المزاج المعتدل فلا يغير

منه شىء وقد يعمل لمن به سوء مزاج حار ولمن به سوء مزاج بارد اما للمعتدل

فيترك على حاله ويجعل ما قرص منه كل قرص مثقال واحد وتعجن الجملة

بثلثة a امثاله عسل وان اريد ان يخمّر ثم يستعمل فيجب ان يعمل b فيه

من الافيون خمسة دراهم ومن الجندبادستر c مساحوقا مثله ولا يستعمل الا بعد

146v ستة اشهر اقله اعنى اذا القى فيه الافيون والجندبادستر واما /من يغلب عليه

سوء مزاج حار فيجب d ان يجعل زعفرانه ومسكه نصف مثقال وينقص منه

الافتيمون ويجعل بدله خمسة دراهم شاهترج واربعة e دراهم سنا مكى ويلقى

فيه الورد وزن f عشرة دراهم بزر بقلة الحمقاء g (ثمينة) [ثمانية] h دراهم طباشير

خمسة دراهم بزر (الحبتى) i [الخس] درهان صندل ثلثة دراهم وتحفظ الادوية

الاخرى بحالها (يقرص) k [يقرص] كما ذكرنا ويعاجن بعسل منزوع الرغوة

بالاستقصاء واما من يغلب عليه سوء مزاج بارد فيجب ان يزاد فى الادوية

قشورl جوز بوّا قشور الاترج عود البلسان زنجبيل فلفل من كل واحد وزن

درهم جندبادستر مثقالان ويقتصر من الكافور على نصف مثقال ويجرى

147r صاحب المزاج الحار ان يتناول نصف الشربة منه مع متقال /طباشير فى رب

التفاح وصاحب المزاج البارد ان يتناول الشربة منه مع وزن (طسوحين) m

[طسوجين] جندبادستر وقد عالجت بعض من يجرى مجرى الملوك عن

المالنخوليا n صعب يضرب الى المانيا وهو للجنون السبعى بهذا (وردت) o [وزدت]

فى النسخة المعتدلة وزن p درهم ياقوت مستقصى (للسحق) q [السحق]

وكان رمانيا نفيسا فانتفع به انتفاعا شديدا بعد اليبس r واما التركيب s

---

a) פינבני.   b) ילקי richtiger!   c) Stets גנדבא (im Texte חנדבא).   d) פינבני.

e) וארבע.   f) מן.   g) Stets אלחממקה.   h) תמאניה.   i) אלקתי.

k) יקרץ.   l) Fehlt.

m) טסוחין.   n) Fehlt.   o) חדת.   p) Fehlt.   q) אלסחק.   r) איאם.

s) אלתדביר.

Kr 43 لخاص باصحاب (الامزاج) [الامزجة] a للحارة التى انما يصيبهم للخفقان وضعف القلب

بسبب b سوء مزاجهم للحار فمنه تركيب بهذه الصفة بزر لخس بزر البطيخ بزر القرع

147v بزر القثاء مقشور من كل واحد وزن خمسة دراهم بزر البقلة للحمقاء | وزن c

اربعة دراهم لؤلؤ بسذ كهرباء سرطان d نهرى محرق ابريسم مقروض e من كل

واحد مثقال رب اللدر مثقال فان لم يوجد فحشب اللدر ثلثة مثاقيل عود

هندى درونج (وربما) [زرنباد] f بهمن ابيض من كل واحد وزن g درهمين

طباشير قاقلة صغار من كل واحد وزن g ثلثة دراهم ورد احمر منزوع الاقماع

يجفف h فى الظل وزن سبعة دراهم زعفران نصف مثقال كافور i مع عشره

مسك محسوق k سحقا شديدا وسدسه عنبر من للجملة مثقال l ونصف

لسان الثور خمسة مثاقيل (يقرص) [يقرص] جملة ذلك على ما بينّا

ويعجن n برّ التفاح ورب السفرجل ورب الرمان اجزاء سوا بمقدار ما

148r يعجنه o ومنه جلاب يتخذ بعصارة لسان الثور | مع مثله عصارة الهندباء واربعة

امثاله عصارة التفاح ومثل للجميع مرتين ماء الورد وسدس ماء اجتمع سكر

طبرزد ويطبخ بالرفق حتى يتقوم p وللجلاب المتخذ بورق البادرنجويية

مطبوخا فى ماء الورد [حتى ياخذ قوته او يلقى عصارته فى ماء الورد] ثلث

وثلثين نافع للجميع من به ضعف q القلب خصوصا ان كان معه لسان الثور

اما اليابس فيطبخ معه فى ماء الورد r [واما] الرطب فيمزج بعصارته فان كان

(المزج) s [المزاج] شديد للحرارة فقل من عصارة البادرنجويية وزيد فَ عصارة

لسان الثور والا اخذا t متساوين.

148 **20.** وينبغى ايضا ان اذكر اعداد الاغذية a. التى يتناول u دائما/فاولها

---

a) אלאמזנה.   b) בחסב.   c) מן.   d) סרטן!

e) מקרץ.   f) זרנבאד   g) Fehlt.   h) מגפף.

i) כאפור מסחוק.   k) Fehlt.   l) ונצף מתקאל.   m) וקרץ.

n) ואלעגן.   o) תעגנה.   p) יתקאום.

q) Folgt: חתי יאכד קותה או ילקי עצארתה פי מא אלורד

r) Folgt וממא.   s) אלמזאג.   t) ואלאנגא.   u) תתנאול.

177

الخبز يعني بجودة القمح ولا يعمل حواري اعني لا يغمس في الماء كما جرت Kr 44 a
العادة لكن يبالغ في نخله حتى لا يبقى فيه شيء من النخالة ويبالغ في
عجنه ويكون ظاهر الملح ظاهر للخمير وتكون الارغفة عادمة اللباب b ويخبز
في التنور او الفرن والتنور افضل .

b. اللحم يقصد ابدا ان يكون اللحم لحم دجاج او فراريج c ويشرب
امراقها دائما فان هـذا الـنـوع من الطير له خصوصية في اصلاح الاخلاط
الفاسدة اي فساد كان وبخاصة الاخلاط السوداوية حتى ان الاطباء ذكروا /
/ان امراق الدجاج تنفع من الجذام d ولا يوخذ من هـذا النوع الا كبيرة 149r
التى اتت (عليه) e [عليها] سنتين ولا صغيرة التى المتخاطئة عليها f غالبة
ولا الهزل (المنه) g [السمنة] ولا الـذى يسمن بالتلقيم h بل السمين الذى لم
يعلف وصورة تدبيره هكذا يطلق الدجاج والفراريج الناهضة في (خرابة) i
[خزانة] متسعة لا يكون فيها مزبلة ولا مرتنة k ويفتقد بالتنظيف l واللمس
الدائم ويلقى لها الطعام الـذى تاكله في اوائل النهار في اوان وهو دقيق
شعير معجون بلبن حليب وان قطع التين اليابس وخلط معه كان افضل m
ولا يجعل لها من الطعام الا قـدر ملو حواصلها فقط ويجعل لها ماء وبعد
ساعات /يبذر لـهـا قمح منقوع بالماء ساعات وفي اخر النهار يقدم لها n ايضا 149v
دقيـق شعير وتين مقطع معجون بلبن فالـدجـاج والفراريج الـتى تدبر o
هكذا نجد p شحمها ابيض لذيذ [ا] وينضج في اسرع وقت ويرطب المزاج جدا
ويعدله q قد تحتّت هذه الاشياء وبان نفعها وان (سأم) r [سئم] مداومة نوع واحد

---

a) וגראת!   b) אלאלבאב!   c) ותשרב.
d) Am Rande: فانه في امراق الدجاج منع للجذام.
e) עליהא.   f) עליה.   g) אלסמנה.
h) באל אלסמין und באל אלתלקים!   i) כّזאנה.
k) מרתّא.   l) באלתנצّיף.   m) אלאפצّל.
n) להם.   o) דבר.   p) תّגّד.
q) קّת!   r) סאה.

Kr 45 فلا بأس ان يوخــذ فى بعض الايام عوضاً منها درّجاً او نبيهوج اما اليمام

فقيه يبس وان كان له خصوصية عجيبة فى تذكية الـذهـن وكذلك للرجل

لا ارى لمولانا به نلونه يمسك الطبع وان تاقتb النفس للحم المواشى فيكون

150r لحم جدى رضيع/وانc لم يكن بد من لحم الضان فى بعض الاوقات فيوخذ

من الخراف ما لم يكمل له حولا نلته قاربه ويوخذ من لحم المقدم خاصّة ولا

يكون مفرط السمن بل من الراعية ولا يوخذ (شيئاً) [شيء] من هذه الا اذا

ملت الدجاج والفراريج.

c. الشراب يستعد منه الابيض اللون ما امكن الرقيـق القوام الطيب

الطعم ان كان فيه قبض يسير (ولا)d [فلا] بأسe الطيب الرائحة الـذىf

التى علبيعلم واحد وقاربهg ويحذر الشديد للحمرة اوh الغليظ القوام او المغير

الرائحة او القديم الشديد المرارة لا يقرب شيءi من هذه الانواع بوجه.

d. الالوان يميل الى كون الالوان حلوة المطعم او يكون فيها (حمضة)k [حموضة]

150v يسيرة او سـذجة وهانا اذكر عـدة الاوانl /ليختار مولانا من ذلك بحسب

وقت وقتm ان مولانا قـد علم اكثرn الاطعمة ولا ينقطع مـن بين يديه

طبيبo يستعان به فى ذلك اولها الدجاج او الفراريج المسلوقةp [المسلوقة]

وايضا المغمومة وايضا المعرقة وايضا المطبوخة (بكر به)q [بكزبرة] خضراء وايضا

التى يلقى فى سليقها رازيانج اخضرr وهذاs اللون يوافق زمان الشتاء وايضا

التى يلقى فى سليقها ماء الليمو او حماضt اترج او ليمو مراكبu وهذه

تصلح لزمان الصيف وايضا المعمولة بلوز وسكر وماء ليمو او خمرv وهـذه

تصلح فى كل زمان وايضا المعمولة بزبيب ولوز ويسير خل وهـذه جيدة فى

---

a) דוראג׳.	b) נאקת!	c) יכוז.	d) פלא.
e) באלטיב.	f) אלחי.	g) או קארבה.	h) Fehlt.
i) שיא.	k) חמוצֹה.	l) והא אנא.	m) בחסב אלוקת.
n) קוי אבֹחֹר.	o) טביבא.	p) אלמסלוקה.	q) באלכסברה.
r) אלכֹצֹרה.	s) והדה.	t) אתרנג׳.	u) מרכב.
v) וכֹמר.			

Kr 46 كل وقت وايضا المعمولة (اسفيدبابج) [باسفيدبابج] a (يسلق) [بسلق] b [بسلق] او بَخَّس

في زمان الصيف وايضا المعمولة بيقطين او باسفاناخ c او يربوز d او باجاص

وهو الذي يسمونه اهل الشام للخوخ e كل هذه جيدة في الصيف ولا بد/

151r من تطييبها (تفرقة) [بقرفة] f ومصطكي وسبل لمنع اضرارها بالمعدة وايضا

المعمولة بالتمر هندي والسكر وايضا المعمولة ببزر الرجلة والسكر وهذه لا

تستعمل الا في الصيف وايضا المعمولة بالورد مربا g وهذه في الشتاء اجود

وايضا المعمولة بفستق وسكر وينبغي ان يضاف اليها يسير ماء ليمو وينبغي

ان لا (يحلو) [يخلو] h لون طعام يوكل في برد الهوى i من الشراب الطيب

المتقدم صفته يقلى به اللحم ان كان لونا مطبوخا k او يلقى في السليق l

ان كان لونا مسلوقا وكذلك الالوان في حر الهوى كلها يلقى فيها في حال

الطبخ قدر عشرين درهما m من الشراب وخمسة دراهم ماء ورد وان كانت/

151v الالوان حامضة فيكون من الشراب عشرين n ومن ماء الورد خمسة ومن الليمو

خمسة وايضا الشوى o ان كانت دجاج فتشوية على السفود على العادة

(وسقا) [وتسقى] p دائما في حال شبيها بالشراب وماء الليمو q او بالشراب وحده

وان (تاقت) [تاقت] النفس لشواء لحوم المواشى فيكون للجدى الرضيع بعد

دهانه s اذا توسط الشى بالشراب ويسير زعفران وكل طعام ينتهيّا ان يجعل

فيه يسير زعفران t لانه دوء قلبى مفرح ولا يكثر منه لان له خصوصية في

اسقاط شهوة الطعام فهذا u ما (حصر) [حضر] المملوك الان من الوان الطعام

التى تصلح لمولانا دامت ايامه.

e. وقد ذكر جالينوس ومن تقدمه من الاطباء شرابا (يسمونه) v [يسمونه]

---

a) באספידבאג׳.	b) בסלק.	c) באספנאך׳.	d) בירבוז.
e) כוך׳.	f) בקרפה.	g) אלמרבה.	h) יכלו.
i) אלהוא.	k) לון מטבוך׳.	l) אלסלק.	m) דרהם.
n) Folgt דרהמא.	o) אלשוא.	p) ...... ותסקי שויהא.	
q) fehlt לרוחאה.	r) נאקת.	s) בעז דה איאם.	t) Folgt יגעל.
u) פהדה.	v) יסמונה.		

180

Kr 47 بلغتهم ادرومالي وكانوا يعملونه من عسل نحل وخمر بيضاء a رقيقة كما كانوا
يعملون السكنجبين من خل وعسل واما المتأخرون فكما عملوا السكنجبين

152r من سكر وخل/كذلك عملوا الادرومالي من سكر وخمر وهذا b شراب فاضل جدا
نافع c لتقوية المعدة والقلب وتحسين الهضم وبسط النفس ويعين على خروج
الفضلتين بمعونة d حسنة جربنا ذلك وجربه غيرنا عدة دفوع.

وصفة عمله ان يوخذ من السكر خمسة ارطال مصرية e ويطبخ كما
يطبخ f الاشربة وتوخذ رغوته ويوخذ له قوام جيد وبعد ذلك يلقى عليه
رطلا واحدا بالمصري من لحم الموصوفة ويعقد شرابا في قوام شراب الورد
وانما ذكر المملوك هذا الشراب مع الاطعمة لانه يجرى مجراها يوخذ دائما
كل يوم g في اوائل النهار في زمان الشتاء بماء حار وفي زمان الصيف بماء بارد

152v ويوخذ منه الثلث اواق والاربعة دفعة لان هذا h الشراب/ليس هو كشراب
السكنجبين وغيره من امثاله لان تلك الاشربة ادوية تحتاج الى تقدير والى
تمييز من يصلح له وهذا h الشراب غذاء فاضل لان السكر بمفرده غذاء وان
كانت فيه (دواية) [دوائية i] يسيرة وكذلك لحم غذاء فاضل بلا شك واعجب ما فيه
قالوا انه لا يضر بالمحرورين وما علة ذلك الا كون بسائطه اغذية جيدة
مألوفة فهذا h قدر ما راى المملوك تقدمته قبل ذكر ترتيب التدبير.

21. فصل في (تدبير) [ترتيب] التدبير لمولانا l بحسب ما شكاه ازال الله
الامه وادام ايامه ولا شك ان هذه المقالة تصل مولانا في استقبال زمان m
الشتاء فلذلك راى المملوك ان يبتدى بصورة التدبير الذي يتدبر به في
برد الهواء n والمملوك يرجو o ان مولانا اذا داوم هذا h التدبير رجعت صحته
لمعتادها في اسرع وقت ان شاء الله تعالى والمملوك لا يعلم عادة مولانا في حال

---

a) ביצה.　　　b) פהדה.　　　c) Fehlt.　　　d) מעונה.

e) מצריא.　　　f) חטבך.　　　g) פי כל יום.　　　h) הדה.

i) דואייא יסירא.　　　k) תרתיב.　　　l) Fehlt, nach שכאה!

m) Fehlt.　　　n) אלהוא.　　　o) ירגוא.

الصحة هل يغتدى a مرة واحدة او يتغدى او يتغدى/ويتعشى فلذلك يذكر التدبير **Kr 48** 153r
بحسب لحالين جميعا b. فاقول يقصد ان يكون الانتباه من النوم ابدا مع
طلوع الشمس او قبل ذلك بقليل ويوخذ حين c ذلك من شراب ادرومالى
اوقيتين او ثلاث ويصبر بعد ذلك ساعة ويركب ولا يزال يركب برفق
ويتدرج d فى اسراع e للحركات حتى تسخن الاعضاء ويتغير النفس فيترك f
حينئذ ويسكن حتى لا يبقى فى ملمسة للجسم والنفس g شىء h ما غيرته
الرياضة وبعد ذلك يغتدى باخذ i الالوان المتقدم ذكرها وياخذ شيئا k من
الفاكهة القابضة كما قد قبل او حبات فستق وزبيب او يسير من للحلواء l
اليابسة او يسير ورد مربا m كل ذلك بحسب ما الفه الان ثم تتكئ/للنوم 153v
ويغنى المغنى بالوتر ويرفع صوته ويجد n نغمته ساعة o ثم يخفض المغنى
صوته على تدريج ويرخى اوتاره p ويلين نغمته حتى يستغرق فى النوم
فيقطع لان قد ذكر الاطباء والفلاسفة ان النوم على هذه الصفة حتى تكون
نغم q الاوتار فى التى تنوم تكسب النفس خلقا حسنا ويبسطها r جدا
ويحسن بذلك تدبيرها للجسد s فاذا انتبه تشاغل بعد ذلك بقية نهاره
بما شاء من قراءة او محاضرة من يوثر محاضرته وهذا هو الاولى اعنى محاضرة
من يوثر محاضرته اما لفضيلته واما لالتذاذ بروئيته t واما لاستخفاف عقله فان
جميع ذلك يبسط النفس (وسعى) [وينفى] u علتها سوء الفكرة فان كان
العادة جارية بتناول غذاء اخر العشاء فيوخد قدر خمسين درهما v من
الشراب الموصوف مزوج بعشرة درام/ماء ورد وعشرين درهما w ماء لسان ثور 154r

---

a) יגתדי ohne diacritische Punkte.

b) Fehlt.   c) חיניד מן שראב   d) ובתדראז.

e) אסרע אלחרכה.   f) פינזל.   g) ואלתנפס.   h) שיא.

i) באחד.   k) שי.   l) אלחלוה.   m) מרבה.

n) ויחד.   o) Fehlt.   p) Folgt אלי אן יסתגרק.

q) תכן יגם.   r) ותבסט.   s) אלי אלגסד.   t) Fehlt.

u) וינפי ענהא.   v) דרהם.   w) Fehlt.

Kr 49 ويوخذ ذلك قليل بعد قليل حتى يحين وقت العشاء فيصبر قدر نصف

ساعة حتى يخرج الشراب عن المعدة وينتعشى على معتاده باخذ a الالوان

المذكورة ثم يحضر المغنى ويشاغله b بالاغانى ساعتين بعد الاكل وينكئ ويامر

المغنى ان يرقف اوتاره ولحانه حتى ينام ويستغرق ويقطع التلاحين c كما

فعل بالنهار وان d كان ثم ليس عشاء ولا يتناول غذاء ثانيا بعد ما تناول

بالنهار فيمزج الشراب على النسبة المتقدمة ولا يزال يتناول منه قليل e بعد

قليل والاوتار تعمل حتى يحين النوم اما بعد ساعتين من الليل او ثلات f

او (اربعة) [اربع] بحسب ما يلذ له المقام ولا (يبالى) [يبالى] عن مقدار ما

يتناوله من الشراب الممزوج كما ذكر اذا ثم ينتعش g ولو تناول منه مائتين

154v (درهما) [درهم]/او ثلث مائة (درها) [درهم] او اكثر من ذلك قليلا فى ليالى الشتاء h لكن

ذلك جيدا ومرطبا للجسم فان كان i جرت العادة بان لا يتناول شيئا على

الشراب الا k بتنقل يسير بحبات فستق محمّص بماء ليمو l او ملح او بيسير

قشر اترج مربّى بسكر او بحب آس محمّص او كزبرة محمّصة فذلك هو الاولى

وان كان جرت i العادة بتناول شيء m من الطعام على الشراب فاجود ما

يتناوله فراريج مشوية على سفود ويكون n من تلك الفراريج التى علفت بما

ذكرنا بدقيق شعير ولبن وتين وحبوب القمح ولان o يظن ان التنقل

بقشر الاترج معتدل بين الحار والبارد وهو دواء قلبى فليعتمد التنقل به فاذا

كان من الغد عند الانتباه من النوم يدبر هذا p التدبير بعينه لا يغير منه

شيئا q/*تنول برد زمان الهوء ويفتقد الحال عند القيام r من النوم فان وجد

عطش كان شرب s السكنجبين الوردى اولى من شرب s ادرومالى وان وجد

---

a) באחד.   b) וישגלה.   c) ללחין.

d) Fehlt bis פימזג, Homoioteleuton, statt פי אלנהאר — באלנהאר.

e) קלילא.   f) תלאתה או ארבעה.   g) ינעם!   h) אלשתי.

i) גראת.   k) Fehlt, ינתקל.   l) לימוא.   m) שיא.

n) ותכן תלך.   o) ולא.   p) הדה.

q) שי טול אלזמאן ברד אלהוא.   r) אלאנתבאה.   s) שראב.

* From here missing in the Jerusalem Hebrew manuscript till Kr 50, 19.

في القارورة فحاجة يسيرة كان شرب a السكنجبين الزبيبى اولى b وان وجد Kr 50

في المعدة امتلاء كان تناول عشرة دراهم من الـورد المربا c وليعلم؟ من ذلك

الاطريفل اولا فان انعاق الطبع او تحجر فليقلل في ما يتناول من الشراب

بالليل او يحذف العشاء ان كان جرت العادة بالعشاء d ويوخذ الشيء الملين

باردا ولا يرتاض في ذلك النهار وقد بيّناه في الفصل الثالث من تلك المقالة

وفي هذه الفصول (كلها) [كلما] f ينبغى التلبيين به والطبيب الحاضر يشير في كل

وقت بما يصلح من تلك الاشياء واما اليوم الـذى g يعوّل فيـه على الحمام

فيشرب h الشراب في اوله كما تقدم ويقلل في (قلة) i [قوة] الرياضة ويقصر k

مدتها ويدخل الحمام باثر الرياضة ويخرج من الحمام ويتناول من الفقاع المعمول

بحب l رمان وسكر وطيب كثير واطراف طيب حارة كالقرنفل والبسباسة او

يتناول شراب ورد (حماض) m [وحماض] بماء لسان ثـور او الشراب n الذى

ركبناه o وذكرناه في الفصل الثالث من تلك المقالة وينام باثر الحمام وقال

جالينوس لم ارم p شيئًا ابلغ في انضاج ما يحتاج الى انضاج وتحليل ما تهيأ

للتحليل من النـوم بعقب الحمام فاذا انتبه تناول الغذاء وتشاغل بقية نهاره

وساعة من الليل بما q ذكرنا فاذا اخذ الطعام في الخروج عن المعدة ياخذ في

تناول ذلك الشراب الممزوج قليلا بعد قليل والمغنى يغنى حتى يستغرق في

النوم على تلك الصورة وليس في تلك [الليلة] r عشاء بوجه ولو جرت العادة

بالعشاء لتناخر الغذاء الى بعد القيام من النوم بعد الحمام واما الوقت الـذى

يعوّل فيـه على الجماع فله s (وقتين) [وقتان] اما/عند انهضام الطعام بعد تناول ذلك 155r

القـدر اليسير من الشراب قبل العشاء او اخر الليل ملال t الامر ان لا يقع

---

a) שראב.	b) אולא.	c) ואלמרבה וארבעה דראהם מן אלאטריפל!	
d) באלעשי.	e) יינא.	f) כלמא.	g) אלחי — בה.
h) פלישרב.	i) קוה.	k) ויקצר.	l) מן חב ריחאן.
m) וחמאץ.	n) ואלשרוב.	o) אלדי רכבנא fehlt.	
p) ארא.	q) כמא.	r) אללילה.	s) כלה.
t) מלאך אלאמר.			

184

هذا a الفعل لا على جوع وخلو معدة ولا على امتلاء المعدة بالطعام وكذا Kr 51
شرب الشراب لا يشرب والطعام فى المعدة لم ينهضم لانه يفاجحه ويخرج
قبل b نضجه ولا والمعدة خالية محتاجة الى تناول الغذاء ·لانه حينئذ يحمى
المزاج ويصلح c ويشيط الاخلاط بل عند اخذ الطعام فى الانهضام وفى كل
جمعة يتناول باكرا d مثقلا واحدا من ذلك المعجون المعتدل المعمول بالياقوت
ولا يرتاض ذلك النهار او من ذلك الاطريفل او من احدى النسخ المذكورة
فى القانون من ادوية المسك ولا سبيل لتناول معجون يكون فيه شىء من
لجندبادستر بوجه /بل بحدف لجندبادستر من كل دواء مسكر يتناوله مولانا 155v
هذا تدبير الزمان الذى يكون الهواء فيه باردا .

واما فى زمان لحرّ f فلا ينبه g من النوم الا بعد ساعة من النهار ويتناول h
الاشربة السكنجبين الوردى والزبيبى والشراب الذى ذكرناه فى الفصل الثالث
من تلك المقالة ويرتاض فى برودة الهواء او يغتدى i بالالوان المائلة الى البرد
وينام طويلا k من سماع الاوتار كما تقدم ولا يتناول من ذلك الشراب الممزوج
الا (قليل) l [قليلا] جدا ولا يسهر بالليل ويقلل لجماع من معتاد الشتاء
ويتناول دواء المسكر البارد الذى ذكرناه عوضا من (يتناول) m [تناول] دواء
الياقوت المعتدل وان اثر شرب شىء من الشراب فليكن n فى اخر النهار
حتى ياخذ منه القدر المذكور وينام فى اول الليل او o فى اخر الساعة
الثانية منه وان اخذ من دواء الياقوت البارد كان /ذلك جيدا p ويكون 156r
الفقاع الذى يشربه بعد لحمام بتمر هندى وسكر مسك وكافور يسير وتلبين
الطبع اذا احتيج اليه بنقيع الراوند والتمر هندى q كما ذكرنا فى الفصل
الثالث من تلك المقالة وكذا r الشراب الذى ركبناه .

---

a) הדה.	b) Fehlt — אלמעדה.	c) ויצרע.	d) Fehlt — מן.
e) Folgt הו.	f) אלחאר.	g) ינתבה.	h) Folgt מן.
i) ויגתדי.	k) סבילה עלי סמע!	l) קלילא.	m) תנאול.
n) פליכן.	o) Fehlt.	p) גיידה.	q) אלהנדי.
r) וכדלך.			

185

وإذا اشتدّ للحرّ a فلا بد من تناول كشك الشعير المدبر فى كل يوم عند **Kr 52**
القيام من النوم قبل الرياضة بساعة عوضا من الاشربة المذكورة او يتناول
عند النوم وينام عليه عوضا مما يشغل المعدة به من غذاء او شراب وصفته
بحسب ما يحتاج اليه مولانا هكذا يوخذ من الشعير المقشور الذى له منذ
حصد ستة اشهر (اربعين) [اربعون] درهًا بزر شاهترج مرضوض وبزر هندباء مرضوص
ولسان ثور من كل واحد اربعة درام بزر خشخاش عراق مرضوص درهمين
صندل ابيض (دهن) b مرضوض درم سنبل ربع درم/زهر شبت نصف درم **156v**
زيت طيب مغربى او شامى اصفر اللون سالم من مرارة الطعم ثلثة درام
يلقى جميع ذلك دفعة واحدة فى c قدر ويلقى على هذا القدر من الماء
الف درم ويرفع على نار فحم حتى يذهب نصف الماء وحينئذ يلقى
عليه ستة درام خل خمر ويتمّ طبخه الى ان يبقى منه دون الربع ويرى
لونه احمر فحينئذ يصفى ويلقى فى صفوه d نصف درم ملح ويتناول وحده
دون شراب وبعد شربه بساعة يلعق ملعقة شراب ليمو e وينبغى لمولانا
ان يعنى بهذا جدا ويقصده ويدمن اعتياده لانه يقاوم يبس لخلط
السوداوى ويعدل الاخلاط (المنحرقة) [المنحرفة] f ويزيل احتراقها ويغلظ
تلك الابخرة المترقية g للقلب والدماغ ويمنع من ترقيها ويبرد المزاج h باعتدال
ويحسن لحال فى كل ما يشكوه مولانا لان ابقراط i يقول فى جملة عدّة k من
فضائل كشك الشعير انه يوصل ما ينبغى الى ما ينبغى ولا يغفل مولانا تعاهده
فى زمان الصيف بوجه الا ان كان الطبع (محتبس) [محتبسا] او حمص l فى المعدة
او احد(ث) [ثت] نفخة فى تحت الشراسيف فانه حينئذ لا ينبغى لمولانا تناوله .

22. والمملوك يعلم ان بجودة ذهن مولانا وحسن m تصوّره يقدر ان يدبر
نفسه كما n ينبغى من تلك المقالة المتقدمة ومن هذه الفصول فكيف اذا كان

---

a) אלחאר.	b) Fehlt.	c) Fehlt — וילקי.	d) צפה.
e) לימוא.	f) אלמנחרפה.	g) אלמרתקיה.	h) Fehlt.
i) בקראט.	k) מא עדה.	l) חבץ.	m) חסן.
n) במא.			

* End of the Jerusalem Hebrew manuscript.

Kr 53 بين يديه من يسترشد بعلمه او يسترفد بأنسه a بالصناعة والله تعالى
الشاهد وكفى به شهيدا لقد كان اعظم امال المملول الاصغر ان يباشر
خدمة مولانا b بجسمه وكلامه لا بقرطاسه وقلمه لكن سوء مزاجه الاصلي وضعف
بنيته الطبيعية ولو في حال الشبوبية ناهيك في حال الهرم حجبت بينه وبين
لذات كثيرة ولا c اقول لذات بل خيرات اعظمها واسناها مباشرة خدمة
مولانا d فالله المشكور على كل لحالات التي تجرى كليّاتها في كليّات الموجودات
(وجزئياتها) [وجزئياتها] e في شخص شخص بحسب مشيئته التابعة بحكمته f التي
لا يدرك الانسان كنهها g ولحمد لله دائما h على كل حال كيف تقلبت الاحوال
ولا ينتقد مولانا على مملوكه الاصغر ما ذكره في مقلته هذه من استعمل
الشراب والاغاني التي i يكره الشرع (كلاهما) [كليهما] ان k المملوك لم (يامن) لم [بامر] l
بان يفعل ذلك وانما ذكر ما تقتضيه صناعته وقد علم المتشرعون كما علم
الاطباء ان لخمر فيها m منافع للناس. ويلزم الطبيب من حيث هو طبيب
ان يخبر n بصورة التدبير النافع كان ذلك حراما o او حلالا والمريض مخبر
ان يفعل او p لا يفعل وان سكت الطبيب عن وصف كل ما ينفع كان حراما
او حلالا فقد غش ولم يبذل النصيحة وقد علم ان الشرع يامر بما ينفع
وينهى عمّا يضر في الدار q الاخرى والطبيب يخبر بما ينفع للجسم وينبه r
على ما يضره في هذه الدار والفرق بين الاوامر الشرعيّة s والمشورات t
الطبيّة ان الشرع يامر بامتثال u ما ينفع في الاجل ويجبر عليه وينهى عن v
ما يضر في الاجل ويعاقب عليه والطبّ يشير بما ينفع ويحذر مّا يضر ولا
يجبر على w ذلك ولا يعاقب على x هذا بل يعرض الامر على المريض على

a) באנסתה.   b) מולאה.   c) לא.   d) ואללה.

e) וגזיאתהא.   f) לחכמתה.   g) כונהא   h) דאימה.

i) אלדי.   k) לאן.   l) יאמר.   m) פיה.

n) יחדר   o) חלאלא או חראמא.   p) לם.

q) דאר.   r) וינהי.   s) ואאמר אלשרע.   t) ואלמשוראת.

u) באמתסאל   v) עמא.   w) עליה.   x) Fehlt בל.

جهة المشورة وهو المخيّر والعلة فى هـذا a بيّنة لان ضرر ما يضر من جهة **Kr 54**
الطبّ ونفع ما ينفع عاجلا أخـذا باليد ولا b يحتاج لجبر ولا عقاب وتلك
الاوامر والنواهى الشرعيّة لا يتبيّن فى هذه الدار ضرها ولا نفعها بل قد c ربما
(تخيّل) [تخيّل d] للجاهل ان كل ما قبل انه e يضر لا يضر وكلما قبل انه نافع لا ينفع
تلونه لا يرى ذلك أخـذا f باليد فلذلك تجبر الشريعة عـلى فعـل للخيرات
وتعاقب على الشرور التى g لا يتبيّن ذلك للخير والشر الا فى الدار الأخرى
كل ذلك احسانا البنا وافضالا علينا ورفقا h (ما) [بنا] لجهلنا ورحمة i [لنا] لضعف
ادراكنا. فهذا k قدر ما رأى المملوك ان يعرضه بين يدى مالك رقه خلد
الله ايامه ورأى مولانا اعلى والسلام l ولواهب m العقل للحمد بـلا نهاية. تمت
المقالة الافصليّة.

---

a) הדה.	b) פלה.	c) קדר במא!!	d) יכיל.
e) Fehlt — נאפע Homoioteleuton!	f) אכّד.		g) אלדי.
h) ורפקנא בנא.	i) Folgt לנא.	k) פהדה.	l) ואסלם.

m) וללה אלחמד ואלמנה אמין

ומן מצנّפאת אלמולוף· נסכّה חבוב ללסעאל אנתפעת בהא ונפעת בהא· והי לב
בזר קתّא ולב בזר בטיך ובזר לשّאש וכזברה אלביר מّו ד' דראהם ערק סוס מגّרוד
מרצّוץ ובזר כתّאن מחمّض مّو עשרה דראהם לסان תّור שאמי ד' דرا' סכّר (נבאת)
[טבדّוד] סתין (דרהם) [דרהמא] تסحق אלאדويה וينכّל ما يمכّن נכّلה מן דّلك וילת
בדהن אללה ويعجّن פי اوקيה תرنجبين קد חّל פי ما راזיانج ويשّل עלי אלאנאר אלي אن
יاכّر קואם אלاשרבّה ويחبّ אמثّاל אלفول نאפع אן شا אللה. نסכّه אلאيارج
פיקרא יوכّر קشر بلסאن וحب بلסאن וסליכّה ואסחق? ودارציני אלצין ومסحכي ואردّر
וזעפראן וסنبל مّو גّو צבر אסקוטרי מثّל אלגّميע תעאلי·

THE MEDIEVAL LATIN TRANSLATIONS

We first present an expanded transcript of the Latin translation of the treatise. This is taken from 4° Inc. s.a. (probably 1477), 1197^t of the Bayerische Staats-Bibliothek. Since the incunable only contains the first eighteen chapters of the treatise, we append an edition of the hitherto unpublished Latin manuscripts, which complete the work.

THE FIRST EIGHTEEN CHAPTERS OF THE TREATISE
EXPANDED TRANSCRIPT OF THE LATIN INCUNABLE

E. D. GOLDSCHMIDT

p.* 65 Peruenerunt ad seruum paruum littere continentes quod debeam de- 130*v*
clarare omnia accidentia illa per capitula et ostendere ipsorum accidentium causas et tempora / innovationis eorum et ponere omnia quae 131*r*
attendit medicus inuestigare et scribere que ea primo oporteat curare
in omni tempore secundum quamlibet ipsorum intentionem et narrare
consimiliter quod medici iusserunt facere in his conditionabiliter et
distincte posuerunt et cognouit seruus ueraciter quod iste littere
de scriptura domini nostri fuerunt absque dubio et iuro perdeum
quod meliores nostri temporis deficiunt a cognitione necessaria in
ordinatione illarum rerum et maxime quia eas non intelligunt ut sciant
eas ordinare et propterea prouideat seruus quod eius responsum ad
regem sit responsum medici ad medicum non responsum ad illum

p. 66 qui non est / de arte postquam diuulgatum est apud regis medicos 131*v*
tractatus domini nostri incognitione illorum accidentium et causarum
eorum et ecce habui notitiam illorum praedictorum accidentium quae
intendit auferre et significauit dominus seruo quod iusserit quilibet
medicus in hoc et mandauit sibi quid scribat ei consilium cuiuslibet
eorum quod propono facere. Qui uero medicorum dixit quod si Chapter 1
flueret sanguis ex uenarum orificiis nunc sicut alio tempore fluxus et
recederent ista accidentia hoc uerum est in quo non est dubium
quoniam sanguis iste qui procedit non est nisi faex sanguinis et eius
superfluitates / quas natura expellit propter malitiam eius per aliquam 132*r*
uiarum crisis. Qui uero dixit apertionem orificiorum uenarum fieri
per sessionem in aquis quae hoc faciunt error est, nec seruus concedit
hoc aliquo modo propter multas causas quas ostendit quarum prima
est quia ille medicine quas faceret uel aque in quibus sederet calide
sunt et necessario calefacerent complexionem et inflamarent humores.
Secunda causa est quia natura quando aperit has uenas competenti
modo aperit eas secundum quod oportet. sed cum aperimus eas cum

p. 67 medicinis ultra quam oporteat aperiuntur et multiplicatur fluxus

---

* The marginal numbering of the pages conforms to the facsimile edition (1931) of the incunable.

sanguinis qui difficilis erit constrictionis quod non accidit quando per
132v se fluit / quamuis fluat multotiens et non ualeat constringi. Tertia est
quoniam iste uene quando aperiuntur per se, exit ex eis quod exire
oportet, natura enim expellit illud ad extremitates et uirtus expulsiua
excitata est ad expellendum. sed quando aperiuntur per has fluit tunc
quod non deberet fluere, et dico uniuersaliter quod nos non oportet
accedere ad hoc artificium nisi loca sint apostemata et augumentetur
eorum dolor ualde, tunc enim oportet eas aperite cum medicina donec
exeat ex eis quod immissum est illuc de sanguine qui locum aparauit
133r [?] et erit actio nostra tunc / quasi ex imitatione nature. sicut in-
conueniens est ante tempus aperire apostemata et educere quod in eo
est sic non conuenit quod faciat dominus noster aliquo modo quod
si sponte contingat fluere sicut multotiens facere consueuit non inten-
dat illud aliquo modo nisi res grauaret multum et ultra mensuram
Chapter 2 restringere. Post hoc uero scripsit dominus quod aliqui medicorum
consuluerunt sumere modicum uini cum aqua buglosse per aliquas
horas post cibum et etiam sumere de hoc eodem parum circa horam p. 68
dormitionis ad profundum eius somnum et significauit mihi supra
hoc quoniam aliqui sunt qui contradicunt huic consilio dicentes non
esse utilem modum ex quo ipsum forte calefacit cerebrum et complexionem et generat uentositates et inflationes. Sed de consilio serui
133v est quod prima intentio / est uerior et etiam si sumat de eo modicum,
scilicet quasi unciam unam orientalis uel circa illud post cibum in hora
digestionis, iuuabit digestionem cibi et addit in expulsione superflui-
tatum per urinam et aufert a sanguine uapores fumosos generantes
hec omnia accidentia existentia nunc et maxime si temperetur cum
lingua bouis uel si infundatur in ipso de lingua bouis quantitas duarum
dragmarum in uncia una esset melius et dilataret animam magis
quando uero medici protulerunt letificatiuum simpliciter uoluerunt
intelligere per illud syrupum de lingua bouis. sed quando ponitur
134r lingua bouis in uino additur ad dilatationem / animae et letificationem
eius et potus uini humettat corpus bona humectatione. Iam Galenus
dixit hoc in regimine sanitatis. Qui uero opinatus est ipsum calefacere
errat quia uinum est non autem medicina et est bonus cibus ualde et
boni cibi neque calefaciunt neque infrigidant, medicina uero ipsa est p. 69
que ualde calefacit et infrigidat. Sed ex uino generatur bonus sanguis
secundum naturam sanguinis naturalis qui est calidus et humidus
limphatum uero absque dubio uentositates generat et possibile gene-
rare tremorem. Narrauit Auenzoar qui singularis fuit in generatione
134v sua et magnus inter nobiles / artis quod uinum limphatum generat illud
si bibatur statim cum limphatur. sed quando limphatur et stat per

unam horam aut plus et deinde biberit illud erit tunc bonum ualde postquam uinositas superat aquositatem et ipsam alterat et rectificat complexionem illud uero quod seruus uult de lingua bouis est cortex radicis eius, non autem uult folium sicut faciunt uiri deacio et Egypto, sic enim uidimus uniuersos senes nobiles facientes in terris hyspanie et in toto occidente similiter utimur corticibus radicis lingue bouis. non autem eius foliis: igitur herbam oportet habere penes ipsum dominum nostrum regem et non distet ab ipsa quia habet proprietatem in dilatatione anime et delet melancoliam et extirpat ipsam ex toto et eorum

p. 70 cuius seruus est expertus et uerificatum apud ipsum in quo non est dubium uinum subtile quando / linphatur cum decima parte aque 135r rosate facit enim animam amplam et non inebriat neque offendit cerebrum et confortat stomacum et auget in omnibus laudabilibus que proprie sunt ipsi uino et ob hoc uult seruus quod apponatur in uncia una orientali de uino dragmas quatuor de aqua rosata et duas dragmas aque lingue bouis et dimissis per quatuor horas uel quasi bibat ipsum postea sed summere ipsum similiter circha horam dormitionis bonum est et oppinio recta est, nam facit profundare sompnum et auferre cogitationes et bonificat digestionem et superfluitates expellit. Concordauerunt medici quod quando complexio est acuta Chapter 3 et ad caliditatem declinat tunc bonum est uti eo quod infrigidat et humectat. / hoc autem uerum est sed comune oportet autem quod 135v distinguatur per capitula et ponatur modus ipsorum uero qui consuluit bibere aquam endiuie cum aqua sandalorum et infusionem tamarindorum prunorum et iuiubarum dicit seruus errorem esse magnum, quia hoc regimen absolutum, cum habet ipsum flegma uictoriam supra

p. 71 complexionem radicalem, non est conueniens aliquo modo maxime pruna et iuiube quia hec debilitant stomacum et nocent et impediunt digestiones et quando stomacus debilitatur et humectatur destruuntur tres digestiones et non ualebit hoc regimen nisi ei / qui abundat colera 136r nigra sed non posuit de significatione colere nigre. Nos uero quod presumpsimus ex predictis signis est generatio fumorum melancolicorum generatorium ex collera rubea generata ex adustione flegmatis abundantis per tempora. Quomodo consulit infusionem reubarbari cum Chapter 4 aqua endiuie per diem quando fuerit intentionis lenificare uentrem. Conueniens est et iam quidem narrauit seruus modum lenificationis nature / cum ipso reubarbaro in capitulo tertio suorum tractatuum 136v qui tractatus sunt in solio domini nostri. Qui uero consuluit introitum Chapter 5 balnei quolibet die tertio et uti exercitio quolibet die et quod ungatur oleo uiolato totum est conueniens et ad hoc loquetur seruus super hoc capitulo distincte et propropius. Qui uero consuluit pecias cum Chapter 6 sandalis epati. Et similiter qui consuluit conmedere citrullum et lactucam et portulacam et spinacias et attriplices, hoc totum est error, p. 72

137r nam hoc remedium confert habentibus febres inflammatiuas / urentes ualde. Et quoniam [?] accidunt in his qui conplexionem habent ualde calidam et in tempore estatis. Et maior error isto est qui iussit potum lactis quoniam considerauit humectationem et dimisit conuersionis facilitatem eius ad quemcunque humorem inuenit in stomaco et non

Chapter 7 considerauit materiam cause egritudinis que est flegma adustum. Et qui signauit summere secaniabin de citoniis post cibum per unam horam, conueniens et utile remedium, bonificat enim digestiones sed

137v adiunctio sua syrupi suci berbene / post dum cibus est in stomaco et etiam si stomacus esset uacuus a cibo non haberet locum ille sucus

Chapter 8 in ista egritudine. Ille autem qui signauit uti syrupo lenificatiuo filii pthomei aut alicuius alterius similiter qui signauit syrupum saltim arabico humati id est acetose uel salsule et pomorum et aque lingue bouis et granorum mirti et seminis trogen, totum hoc est conueniens,

138r sed adiungere cum hoc psilium / non uidetur conueniens in hoc loco, non enim uideo in ipso bonum regimen in hac discrasia et conplexione. p. 73

Chapter 9 Qui uero signauit sumere aquam ordei cum papuere et semine cori esse mirabile in rectificando sonnum et quasi cum habet aquam ordei uirtutem humectationis breuem sonnum confortabit ipsam semen cori et mirabilius hoc est eius qui dixit summere pruna post aquam ordei. ego quidem non puto secundum istos medicos quod sit aliquod membrorum corporis magis proprium quam stomacus. Ille uero

138v qui non curat, si debilitetur stomacus / uel non debilitetur, et si accipiat in ipso impedimentum uel non cum possibile sit eis confiteri nobilitatem stomaci et multitudinem utilitatum suarum quapropter oportet adhyberi curam circa ipsum continuo. et ideo fecit super ipsum nobilior medicorum tractatum Verum tamen hoc responsum apud illos confortat stomacum eius digestionem bonificat et exiccat eius humiditatem et eius uiscositatem incidit que generantur ex flegmate quod non desinit generari in ipso quotidie et subtiliat quod grossum est in ipso. et est illud regimine cuius memoria precessit apud eos quod est aqua ordei cum semine corticis proprius incipiendo post illud cum

139r primo nimis redarguit / ergo seruus quod redarguendum in hoc casu

Chapter 10 ut caueat dominus et non indigeat generaliter dicto. Sumere autem p, 74 poma et citonia et sumere grana granatorum post cibum consulendum est omnibus hominibus in regimine sanitatis nec in hoc est additio pertinens huic egritudini. Quod uero signatum fuit de sumptione pitartimi id est coriandorum habet in se naturam in grossandi uapores et prohibendi eos ascendere. quod quidem uerum est nihilhominus

oportet quod sumatur cum medicinis sicut sunt / grana suffufur et   139*v*
huius modi uel coquatur cum medicina sed sumere coriandrum solum
post cibum, et si non inducat uomitum, generat pustulas absque
dubio et corrumpit cibum. Sumere autem semen portulace cum
zucharo aliquibus temporibus preter quod cum cibo bonum est et
etiam si misceretur cum ipso cibo non lederet in eo quod regit et confortat cor. Et signauit dominus noster quoniam medici signauerunt   Chapter 11
ei uti mesmes .i. crisomilis et piris et citoniis cum cibo uuis et mel-
lonibus et granatis et ante hoc non cognouit seruus / intentionem huius   140*r*
signationis utrum fuerit propter necessitatem appetitus et consuetudinis sumendi, et de fructibus, quod quidem conuenit sumere de ipsis
ante commestionem quod lenificet naturam, post conmestionem uero
p. 75   quod constringit et coadunat, sicut sunt pira citonia et poma, hoc
est conueniens quod si intendit dicere quod usus istorum fructuum
conferat huic discrasie error est. nam fructus omnes humidi sunt mali
ct sanis et egris quaniam accipiuntur per uiam cibi, et maxime me-
lones et mesmes que dicuntur bacohoc in hispania omnes sunt mali
pro multitudine alterationis ipsorum ad quemcumque malorum humorum existentium in corpore: / similiter et persica pexima, sunt   140*v*
enim materia malarum febrium et fraudulentarum. Et Galenus dixit
quod a die aqua manum abstraxit a commestione fructuum humido-
rum non percepit febrem usque in finem dierum suorum, et prolon-
gauit sermonem suum super hoc per modum corruptionis humorum,
sicut scriptum est in eius tractatu propter quod necesse est quod re-
linquat dominus noster omnes fructus humidos toto eius posse: qui   Chapter 12
uero consuluit relinquere omnes carnes uenationis et carnes que
uocantur adir et melangranas dixit bene. nam omnia hec uigent in
illud de quo conqueritur dominus ex ipsis accidentibus. Similiter
quoque qui consuluit exercitium omni die, conuenienter dixit. Simi-
p. 76   liter qui prohibuit ipsum accedere ad regiones calidas / dissoluunt enim   141*r*
in homine uapores. scilicet ascendentes ad superficiem corporis dum
frigidi et humidi sunt. Vaporibus enim illis ascendentibus qui reso-
luuntur ex sanguine grosso et turbido ille regiones addunt in grossi-
tudinem et ustionem sanguinis et eius uapores multiplicant. quando
uero perficietur sanitas domini in adiutorio dei poterit moueri et ire ad
quecunque eius desideria deus adimpleuerit tam in hoc seculo quam
in futuro. Non uidetur seruo quod dominus euacuet corpus eius cum   Chapter 13
lapide lazuli uel cum lapide armeno. non cum lapide lazuli propter
eius uehementia cum lapide uero armeno quia non cognoscitur et
iam intulit in ipso dubietatem nobilis medicorum et plurimi ita quod
non est iste qui nuncupatur hoc nomine. eodum modo uidetur seruo

141v esse conueniens / cauere sibi dominum ab administratione medicinarum laxatiuarum fortium et sit contentus de reubarbaro uel aqua
casei et cima methi et his similibus hec omnia conuenientia sunt. nec
uidetur seruo facere infusionem persicam nec aquam melonum in eo
quod nocet stomaco non enim est id de quo conqueritur dominus p. 77
noster ex ipsis egritudinibus inflammatio neque sitis. nec etiam
uidetur seruuo quod utatur multum de nenuphare quia ingrossat
sanguinem et debilitat stomacum. hec non sunt bona nisi patientibus
febres acutas, sicut narrauit seruus. nec uidetur seruo administratio /
142r decoctionis epithimi quia molestat et exsiccat quod infundatur epithimum et ponatur in aqua eius uncia .i. de aqua casei et accipiat bis uel
ter tempore ueris. et semel uel bis in hyeme esset bonum et inter
quamlibet uicem sit spatium .xv. dierum et frigetur epithimum cum
oleo amigdalarum quod ligetur in petia panni lini subtilis et ampli-
Chapter 14 deinde infundat ipsum per noctem in aqua casei. Et signauit dominus
noster quod, quando flebotomatur, exibat sanguis grossus quasi
splen, et dixerunt medici supra ista flobotomia[1] quando apparet se-
142v cundum tempus plenitudo ex qua / sequitur necessario educere et
auferre de sanguine secundum id. sed quod oportet considerare super-
est subtiliare sanguinem et rectificare complexionem epatis ut gene-
ret bonum sanguinem. hoc quidem determinauit seruus in precedenti
143r 5 tractatu quod hoc fiat cum syrupis predictis.[2] / Qui uero signauit potum p. 78
Chapter 16 syrupi letificatiui et electuarium in quo sint lapides pretiosi ut granata
smaragdi et argentum et aurum, totum hoc bonum est et utile ualde,
quia iste sunt medicine cordiales iuuatiue sua proprietate. scilicet
forma specifica que quidem est tota eorum essentia. id est substantia
Chapter 17 non simplex qualitas. Qui uero signauit domino de usu administratio-
nis lingue bouis et nenufaris et cum toto hoc non fuit extirpata radix
discrasie. Causa huius est frequens usus nam medicine conuertuntur
in nutrimentum quando continuo fiunt quia natura recolligit eas ad
se et diligit propter quod non potest habere manifestam operationem
quia quasi nutrimentum efficitur uel proprie nutrimentum. et Galenus
quidem dixit quod huius debiles medicine si recipiantur per unam
septimanam continuo perditur earum operatio medicinalis et non
143v apparebit in eis deinde manifestus effectus. / et propter hoc bonum
est transferri de medicina in medicinam et relicta prima medicina
Chapter 18 per dies aliquos tunc poterit redire ad ipsam. Qui autem signauit
de diminutione coytus preter consuetudinem, sic faciendum est

---

[1] *Should read* flebotomia (*see* Du Cange iii 524)
[2] Chapter 15 is missing in the latin version.

p. 79 quoniam maxima resultat utilitas in eius dimissione. balneum quoque [?] non est renuendum aliquo modo non in tempore coytus
non in tempore quietis et quod sumpsit secundum consuetudinem
bonus et perfectus. Probatio uero huius est quia fumi melancolici non
molestant cerebrum nec alterant eius modum sed molestant cor tan-
tum. eius uero quod sentit dominus debilitatis post saporem[3] id est
exercitium / causa huius est dimissio et interpollatio. Nam si gradatim
rediret ad ipsum paulatim percipiet in fine eius fortitudinem et leti-
tiam, que solent resulutare post quodlibet exercitium debite rectum.

Laus deo et Marie uirgini.

Imprexum Florentie,
apud Sanctum
Iacobum de
Ripolis.

---

[3] Ms. Friedenwald: laboram; Ms. Vatican: soporem; Ms. Vienna: *missing*.

THE HITHERTO UNPUBLISHED PART OF THE LATIN TEXT

F. KLEIN-FRANKE

INTRODUCTION TO THE MANUSCRIPT: LIBER DE CAUSIS ACCIDENTIUM

The Latin version of the *Kitāb al-aʿrāḍ* of Maimonides has previously only been printed to the end of Chapter XVIII. In the present work an edition of the subsequent chapters until the end of the treatise is presented for the first time. The translator is Johannes Capuensis (fl. 1262–1278), who also translated the *Regimen Sanitatis* of the same author, of which the *Liber de causis accidentium* was sometimes erroneously held to be a part. Steinschneider has dealt with the history and the transmission of this treatise (Steinschneider, HÜ pp. 773–4). The present critical edition is based upon the first two Latin manuscripts noted above, of which Steinschneider knew only V.

The Latin text established here has been checked against the Hebrew text (E), and a double page has been found to be missing between E fol. 155*r* and fol. 155*v*. It has also been collated with the Arabic text edited by Kroner. Following the completion of this work, a reproduction of Latin MS. Palat. 1298 from the Vatican Library was received. This, however, did not yield new readings, and because it is similar to H it did not require further consideration.

Manuscripts H and V, which have been described by Bar-Sela and others (1964), are of the same recension, but differ from one another in a number of readings and peculiarities, examples of which will be given below. In both cases the text is well preserved and had to be conjectured in very few places.

Because this edition is intended not only for scholars of medieval Latin but also for physicians and others who are interested in the history of medicine, the Latin text has been rendered as legible as possible, the numerous and complex abbreviations have been written out in full, and (except in the critical apparatus) the spelling

Sigla: H = Latin MS. Fr. 5₇1–6 (Accidents: fol. 195*v*–199*r*) of the Friedenwald Collection the Hebrew University, Jerusalem

      V = Latin MS. 5306 (Accidents: fol. 11*v*–19*r*) of the Österreichische National-bibliothek, Vienna

      R = Latin MS. Biblioteca Apostolica Vaticana, Palat. Lat. 1298

      E = Hebrew MS. 3941, The Jewish National and University Library, Jerusalem

commonly used in medieval manuscripts has been replaced by the classical spelling, thereby avoiding ambiguity. Thus where medieval "e" stands for classical "ae" the latter has been substituted, as epistulae instead of epistule (200,1); in the same way indii replaces yndij (201, 13), nihil stands for nichil (207, 3), urit for hurit (209, 26), and so on. The same procedure has been applied to words which are uncommon even in medieval spelling and thus do not even appear in specialized dictionaries, such as that of Du Cange. In such a case, the irregular form is noted in the critical apparatus as a "peculiar error," special to the manuscript. Some of these are instructive with regard to the pronunciation of Latin in the Middle Ages: for example, lingni instead of ligni (202, 15), angliculi instead of agniculi (204, 9).

V is much more elaborate than H. The scribe of H generally inserts one consonant where two are required, as in galinarum (203, 10), molifiet (207, 11), percusione (207, 12), surectionem (208, 20 and 209, 17), pasulis (208, 24); but dillatationem (206, 1) and accetositatis (204, 19). Melanconico (203, 13 and 211, 9) and exiscatorum (202, 16) may be vernacular forms. Spellings such as carbae (201, 5) and bugolossae (201, 5) have been eliminated. That the scribe of H was not well versed in the Latin language can be seen from the fact that he writes vincitur (201, 22), asetur . . . cum . . . spico (205, 14), sanantibus (208, 2), liniri (209, 2), dissolve (209, 11), paratum (210, 20), legunt (212, 7), elligat (212, 19), and so on. He sometimes prefers a simple form, such as surexerit (209, 17) instead of resurrectionem, hurit (209, 26), instead of adhurit, and so on. The place left for the insertion of the initial letters by the rubrificator has usually been left empty. However, different as they are, the two manuscripts complement one another to a great extent.

The Final Chapters of the Treatise

AN EDITION BASED ON MEDIEVAL MANUSCRIPTS

Postquam respondit servus super quosdam capitulorum epistulae 1
honorabilis secundum eius mandatum, poterit ipse congregare tractatum et respondere per alia capitula quale oportet esse regimen
domini nostri secundum illa accidentia nunc in ipso repperta et hoc
tam in his quae determinata sunt in his quae posita sunt in hac epistula, 5
quae ex his quae memorata sunt in illo tractatu qui quidem sunt
144v speciales sermones, sed non communes. Et antequam / incipiam hoc
capitulum dico, quod oportet esse in / palacio domini nostri post R197a
syropos et triferas quas memoravit servus in capitulo tertio eius
praecedentis tractatus duo electuaria, quorum unum est medicina 10
frigida de musco facto, cuiusque experti sunt senes artis medicinae
in usu eorum et inventa est in ipso operatio mirabilis valde, donec
volunt, quod aliud intret in loco eius et vocant ipsum electuarium, et
est medicina, quam scripsit Alrasi in libro suo, quem expellit Nocumenta Ciborum. Cuius compositio ad textam est haec: recipe rosa- 15
rum pistarum spodii coriandri sicci chadebe an partem unam et musci
145r boni et puri partem sextam et accipiatur / de zuccaro tabarzet et
dissolvatur in succo pomorum acrium expresso et colato et decoquetur,
donec fiat ad modum mellius et ponatur in foliis citri et conficiatur
cum eo medicina et utatur ea, qui patitur hoc accidens, quum est 20
medicina sublimis in confortatione cordis cum caliditate. Medicina
electuarium aliacut, quod discripsit Avicenna in suo divulgato tractatu, quem appellant De Medicaminibus Cordialibus et dixit, quam
est trium discriptionum prima quidem est frigida, altera calida, tertia
temperata. Quod autem videtur / servo super his est, ut dominus 25 V14a

5 ex his quae iam determinata sunt ex his quae posita sunt H   7 sed non communes om. H
9 siropos V   eius om. V   13 et appellant ipsum H   14 in marg. V: Electuarium cordiale;
in marg. H: Electuarium   16 partis unius V   17 zucharo H   18 in succo malorum H
collato V   coquatur H   19 admodum V   21 fortatione V   22 in marg. V: Electuarium secundum; in marg H: secundum Electuarium est om. H   electuarium H   scripsit V   24 quem
appellant om. V   medicaminibus om. V   25 dominus om. H

XVI

XVII

XVIII

XIX

Facsimile of the Latin translation
MS. Cod. Lat. 5306
Oesterreichische Nationalbibliothek, Vienna

Facsimile of the Latin translation
MS. Friedenwald 572
Jewish National and University Library, Jerusalem

Facsimile of the Latin translation
MS. Palat. Lat. 1298
Biblioteca Apostolica Vaticana, Rome

1 utatur temperata. Haec est discriptio ad tertiam: Inquit ipse dis-
H196d criptio / autem optima, cuius expertus sum, et est electuarium et
trocisci, de qua addidi et diminui secundum quaslibet complexiones,
cuius / iuvamentum et confortatio cordis est maxima; eius modus 145v
5 hic est: recipe margaritarum, carabi, coralli an drachm. 1½, buglossae dr. 5, setae crudae incisae, caneriorum fluvialium an dr. 1½,
auri limati dr. 2, seminis badromomae et melissae tres uncias, been
albi et rubri, ligni aloes, lapis armeni, lapis lazuli loti, masticis,
cassiae, cinamomi, croci, cardamomi maioris, cubebarum an dr. 1,
10 epithimi an aur. 2½, sticados dr. 3, zedoariae aur. 1, et si non invenia-
tur, ponatur loco eius zedoariae aur. 2, seminis endiviae dr. 5, seminis
citrullorum dr. 4, mannae dr. 8, rosarum rubearum dr. 4, / musci aur. 146r
2, camforae aur. 2, ambrae aur. 1, spicae folii indi dr. 2, fiant trocisci
et conficiantur cum melle et ambae fiant secundum complexionem
15 temperatam et non mutetur de eis quidcumque et administretur
habenti malam complexionem. Mediocris vero dimittatur secundum
sui compositionem ac complexionem et sit quilibet trociscus unius
unciae et conficiatur totum cum tribus partibus mellis. Et si volunt
miscere et postea administrare, oportet quod ponatur in ipso de
20 epithimo dr. 5 et de castoreo pulverisato eandem quantitudinem et
non ponatur de ipso nisi post menses sex ad minimum, si quid ponat-
⟨ur de⟩ epithimo ⟨et⟩ castore⟨o⟩. Sed / ille, in quo vincit malioritas 146v
complexionis calidae, oportet quod sit crocus et muscus eius an
dimidiae drachmae et subtrahat deinde epithimum et loco eius ponat
25 fumae terrae dr. 5, spodii dr. 4, sandalis dr. 3; conservetur haec
medicina secundum modum eius et fiant trocisci sicut diximus et
sint confecti cum melle despumato bene. Sed illi, in quo dominatur
complexio frigida, oportet quod addatur illis medicamentis corticis
nucum orientalium, corticum citri carpobalsami drr., piperis an dr. 1

---

1 descriptio rerum H   descriptio V   2 autem om. V   3 trocisi H   4 magna H   et eius V
5 in marg. V: Electuarium bonum valde; carabae V; carbae H bugolossae H   7 badro-
borum H (arab.: badrug); quatuor uncias et tres drachmas V ben H   8 loti om. H   9 cassias
lineae H   cubebarum añ aur. 1 H   10 zedoarae H; et si . . . zedoarae dr. 2 om. V   12 citroli H
13 camfori H aur. 2 om. V yndij H trocisi H   15 quidcumque. Et V   17 et quilibet trociscus qui fiet ex eo fiat unciae unius H   18 Et si folunt administrare et postea   20 pulve-
rizato H   quantitudinem om. V   21 si de epithimo et castore V; si quid ponat epithimo
castore H   22 vincitur V   malia V   24 sed subtrahat tamen V deinde om. V   ponat
om. V   26 et fiat trociscus H   27 conficiatur H spumato H ille, in quo V; illi, quo H
29 carpobalsami unce.

et casto / rei dr. 2. et non ponatur in ea camfora nisi / aur. ½. Et ^{V14b}
sufficit habenti complexionem calidam accipere de eo medicina ^{R197b}
147r acceptionem aur. ½ spodii cum rob de pomis et habens complexionem
frigidam sumat de eo cum scrupulo uno castorei. Et ego quidem curavi
quendam, qui erat magnus dominus et regebat se regimine principum 5
et regum dominorum, ab aegritudine scilicet fatuitate cum praedicto
et addidi in hac discriptione mediocri dr. 1 iacutorum tritorum valde et
erat granata sublima et carissima et recepit maximum iuvamentum
propter hoc post paucos dies. / Compositio vero propria habentibus ^{H197a}
complexionem calidam, quibus accidit sincopis et cordis debilitas causa 10
maliciae complexionis cordis: recipe seminis lactucarum, seminis atri-
147v plicis, seminis citrulli excorticati an dr. 5, seminis portulacae / dr. 4,
margaritarum, corallorum, carabi, cancrorum fluvialium ustorum, setae
incisae an aur. 1, radicis capparorum aur. 1 et si non invenitur, ponatur
loco eius ligni aloes, zedoariae, been albi an dr. 2, spodii, cardamomi 15
minoris an dr. 3, rosarum rubearum in umbra exiccatarum dr. 7,
croci aur. 1, camforae tritae cum decima parte ambrae sui musci
triti bona contricatione et sexta eius parte ambrae omne aur. 1½,
linguae bovis aur. 5; fiant ex eis trocisci cum rob malorum sicut
diximus et cum rob de cydoneis et rob de granatis an partes aequales, 20
quod sufficiat ad incorporandum; ex ipso Julep sumat cum succo
148r buglossae et / cum tantundem succi endiviae et quadruplico eius succi
malorum et duplo omnium aquae rosarae et sexta parte eius, quod
est de zuccaro tabarzet et coquatur totum suaviter, donec habeat
modum debitum. Julep vero factum cum foliis basiliconis decocti cum 25
aqua rosata quousque recipiat virtutem eius, vel ponatur succus
eius in aqua rosarum tertia parte et duabus tertiis iuvat omnem ha-
bentem debilitatem / cordis imprimis et quando fuerit cum eo bug- ^{V14c}
lossa; in sicca complexione coquatur cum aqua rosata, in humida

---

1 11 non om. H   in ea om. H   de camfora H   2 sufficiat H   accipere acceptionem medicinam V; de eo om V   4 castorei H   5 quendam] magnum dominum [et regebat se V   6 et
regum dominorum om. H   ab aegritudine] fatuitatis V   7 addici V   descriptione V   iacut
scilicet lapides triti valde H   8 sublimia H   et carissima om. V   magnum V   9 post
hos per paucos dies H   vero om. V   10 malam [complexionum calidam V   debilitas cordis H
11 complexionum [cordis], quae resultat ex iis ista est compositio H   lactucae H   12 citroli H
13 setae combustae H   aur. 4 V   14 caparis H   15 lingni V   16 rorum V   rubearum
om. V   exiscatorum H   17 camphorae H   19 bovis dr. 5 H   ex hijs H   20 citoniis HV
aequales quam tenet sufficiat ad conficiendum H   21 accipiat H   suco bugolossae H   22 qua-
druplici H   23 sextam partem H   25 modum om. V   27 rosaria H   28 fuerit omni eo H
28 bugolossa H

1 vero cum succo eius; si vero complexio fuerit vehementis caliditatis, cum modico succo basiliconis et adde de succo buglossae an partes aequales.

Capitulum de cibariis — Et oportet, ut ponam genera ciborum, quibus
5 uti / , et primum panis de bona farina; et non faciat panem nobilem, 148v quem non infundat ipsum in aqua sicut consuevit fieri, sed excedat in separatione furfuris ex eo et excedat in eius comparatione et percipiatur sal in ipso et similiter fermentum et sint placentulae privatae micis et coquatur in furno, quia melior erit.

10 Capitulum de carnibus — Carnes vero sufficit, quod sint semper gallinarum vel pullorum carnes et bibat semper brodia earum, quoniam hoc genus avium habet proprietatem in rectificando complexiones humorum melancolicorum, donec dixerint medici, / quod brodia 149r gallinarum conferunt leprae; et non accipiatur de hoc genere nec
15 multum antiqua, quae praeterierit duos annos, nec parva, in qua
R197c abundet mucilla generositas, nec multum / macilenta nec multum pinguis. Modus autem nutricationis ipsarum sic est: solvantur gallinae magnae cum parvis in domo una ampla, in qua non sit stercus
H197b nec sordicies / et saepe mundificetur locus ubi sunt, et ponatur cibus
20 quem debent accipere in primo diei in aliquis vasis, et sit cibus, quem ponet ibi, farina ordei distemperata cum lacte, et misceantur cum ipsa frustra caricarum, quoniam melius est, quod non adminstretur ei de cibo nisi, qui melior et competentior est, et adminstretur illis de aqua; post autem aliquas horas / adminstretur illis de farina distempe- 149v
25 rata cum aqua per aliquas horas. In fine autem diei paeoccupet eas etiam farina ordei et frustis caricarum distemperatis cum lacte. Iuvenes enim pingues harum gallinarum et pullorum albam et dul-
V14d cem / habent carnem et digestibilem in stomacho in modica hora et

1 vel (pro vero) V; sive (duabus postremis litteris deletis) H   vero om. H   2 succi H; et om. V
bugolossae H   3 aquales V   4 Capitulum de cibariis om. V   in marg. V: de pane   quod
(pro ut) H   5 uti. Et H   7 a separatione H   reparatione V   10 in marg. V: de carnibus
Arnes H   galinarum H   11 et (pro vel) H   broda H   12 in rectificatione humorum
melanconicorum H   14 galinarum confert laesis H   15 magna (pro antiqua) H   16 ha-
bundet muscila H   macilentes H   17 pingues H   vero (pro autem) H   ipsarum nutricationis H   18 galinae parvae cum magnis H   20 quem ponet ibi om. V   21 misceatur H
22 et (pro quod) H   23 eis H   qui melior est et contemptior est H   administret H   illis
om. V   24 farinam infusam in aquam H   25 vero (pro autem) H   etiam eas V   26 frus
tris H   27 Invenies enim pinguedinem harum galinarum et pullorum albam et dulcem digestibilem H

humectat cerebum nimis et rectificat ipsum. Ista quidem rectificata sit　1
et rectificatum est ipsorum iuvamentum. Quod si habuerit taedium,
uti eius utatur loco earum carnibus fasianorum, et renues turtures
vero retinent siccitatem, licet habeant mirabilem proprietatem in
rectificatione intellectus et in clarificatione eius. Similiter starnae　5
non videntur nobis propter differentiam, quia ipsae constringunt
ventrem. Quod si animus tuus dilexerit ad carnes accedere quadru-
150r pedum, sint carnes edi lactantis. / Similiter cum non sit dubium
animos omnes declinare ad carnes ovinas, sint agni annualis vel
circa illud et accipiat anteriores solum et partis anterioris, et non sit　10
multum pinguis et sit ex pascentibus, et non utatur istis nisi post
eius fastidium gallinarum et pullorum.

Capitulum de vino — Vinum vero exhibeatur album in colore,
quantumcumque potens sit et quod sit subtile et boni saporis. Et si
habuerit aliquid coadunationis, non est nisi bonum et non malum　15
odiferum, quod praeterierit annum vel circa; et caveat a vino rubeo
valde et a grosso in substantia et alterata in colore aut veteri et amaro
nec praesumat de aliquo istorum generum aliquando. Fercula vero
declinent ad dulcem saporem vel quod habeant aliquid acetositatis
150v vel multum. Ego autem narrabo fercula / , ex quibus eligat dominus　20
secundum temperantiam, postquam dominus meus novit virtutes
cibariorum et non est absque medico, a quo semper accipiat consilium.
Imprimis est pullae et pulli masculi parvuli, elixati in aqua cum
coriandro humido. Et scilicet potest fieri cum feniculo, et hoc epulum
est utile tempore hiemali. Et iam illud, in cuius decoctione ponitur　25
succus limonum vel acetositas citri aut limonum mixtim, et hoc erit
utile tempore aestatis. Quae vero fiunt cum amigdalis et zuccaro et
succo limonum, sunt bona omni tempore. Scilicet quae fiunt / cum　H197c
passulis et amigdalis, sunt bona omni tempore. Et quae fiunt / in aqua　V15a

1 rectificant ipsum ita, quod rectificatum est ipsorum iuvamentum V   3 tehug (pro renues) H
4 siccitates H   5 rectificacatione V   proprietatem in clarificatione intellectus H   6 nobis...
constringunt om. V   7 declinaverit (pro dilexerit) H   8 accedere om. H   9 angliculi
(pro annualis) H   10 anteriores solum et om. H   exparte anteriori solum H   12 eius
om. V   13 in marg. V: de vino   Inum H   administretur H   14 potens V   16 circa.
est V   cavea V   17 crosso H   veteri valde H   18 generum aliquo modo V   19 accetositatis H; acotositatis V   20 et (pro vel) V   elligat H   21 temperantias H   22 recipiat H
23 masculi < arab.: maslūqa   parvuli om. H   25 yemali HV   iam om. H   26 acce-
tositas H   27 zuccario V; zucaro H   28 suco H   et scilicet... tempore om. V   et]
scilicet [quae V   29cum aqua V

1 sola cum bletis aut lactucis, tempore aestatis, aut cum prunis; omnia
haec sunt bona in aestate; / et omnino bonum / est ponere in ferculis 151r
de speciebus sicut cinamomo, mastice et spica et huius similibus.
R197d Nam prohibent nocumentum ferculi in stomacho. Et quae / fiunt
5 etiam cum semine portulacae et zuccaro, in aestate. Tum et ea, quae
fiunt cum zuccaro et cum rosis, meliora sunt in hieme. Et ea, quae
fiunt cum festuce et zuccaro addito eis modico succo limonis. Et
oportet, quod non sit aliquid ferculum, quod comedit in hieme absque
appositione boni vini. Et modus huius ferculi hic est: coquantur
10 carnes in brodio de bletis et similibus, et secundum diversitatem
aeris apponatur de vino circa viginti drachmas et aqua rosarum quinque drachmas. Quando / fercula erunt acetosa et sit quantitas vini vi- 151v
ginti drachmae et aquae rosatae quinque drachmae. Assata vero si fuerit
gallina, assetur cum spica sicut consuetudo est et inbibatur semper
15 dum assatur cum vino et succo limonum. Quod si animus declinaverit
ad assatum carnium quadrupedum, sint carnes edi lactantis, quae
post mediam assationem inbibantur vino et modico croci et quolibet
cibario, in quo ponitur aliquid croci bonum est, quoniam est de medicinis cordis, qua laetificat ipsum; sed non sumat de eo magnam
20 quantitatem. Nam eius proprietas est auferre appetitum cibi. Hoc
est, quod pervenit ad manum meam de bonis ferculis pro domino
nostro rege, cuius deus prolonget dies. Galenus vero et qui fuerunt
ante ipsum medicorum posuerunt sirupum dictum ydromel, qui est
de melle et vino albo et subtili, sicut fit secaniabim de acetoet melle.
25 Et veluti vero sicut faciebant / secaniabim ex zucharo et aceto, ita fa- 152r
ciebant ydromel atque mellicratum ex zucharo et vino. Tale enim
vinum nobile est ad confortandum stomachum et cor et rectificandam

1 latucis H   prunijs H   4 in om. H   5 zuccario V; zucaro H   6 cum om. H; rosato H
yeme HV   7 existucis (pro: cum festuce) V   zuccario V; zucaro H   succo om. H
limonumV   8 ferculum] cibi H   yeme HV   9 appositioni V   est hic H;   10 cum brodio H   velcum similibus H   11 et quinque drachmas de aqua rosata H   12 Quando ...
quinque dr. (pag. sequ.) om. H   12 accetosa H   13 Assatum H   14 galina H   asetur H
spico H   sicut commune et consuetudo est. Et V   continue (pro semper) V   15 cum
(pro dum) V   16 assatis V   qui H   17 unguatur cum vino H   et in quolibet H
18 si (pro: in quo) V   de croco H   19 utatur de eo in magna quantitate H   20 aufferre H
et hoc V   22 Galienus V   quidem (pro vero) H   23 medicorum om. V   syrupum H
quod H   24 albo et om. V   fit om. V   de vino et aceto V   25 Et ... aceto om. V
faciebat V   26 mellicratum om. H   ex vino et zuccario V   27 corpus, ad confortandam
digestionem V

digestionem et dilatationem animae et iuvat ad educendum ambas   1
superfluitates optimo iuvamento, cuius experti sumus et alii nostri ante-
cessores. / Et modus eius est, quod accipiatur ex zuccaro quinque libr.   V15b
ad lb. aegyptii et coquatur ad modum sirupi et auferatur eius spuma
et acquiratur ei bonus modus, deinde eiciatur super ipsum de vino   5
bono praedicto lb. unam de aegypto et fiat inde sirupus ad modum
sirupi rosati. Servus autem posuit hunc sirupum cum cibariis, quia
habet hanc considerationem cum eis et accipiatur ex eo continuo
omni die in primo diei tempore frigoris / cum aqua calida, in aestate   H197d
vero cum frigida; et dosis eius est tres unciae vel quatuor vice qualibet,   10
152v   quia hoc vinum / non est sicut sirupus secaniabin vel alii consimiles.
Nam illi sirupi sunt medicinae et indigent quantitate et distinctione
secundum complexionem hominis, cui convenit. Sed hoc vinum est
cibus nobilis, nam zuccarum per se cibus est, quamvis obtineat partem
medicinae. Similiter vinum cibus nobilis est absque dubio; et quod   15
magis mirabile dixerunt de vino, est, quoniam non laedit calidos
natura. Et causa huius non est nisi quia eius simplicia sunt bonum
nutrimentum et amabile. Et hoc est, quod visum est servo; praepo-
nere ante memorationem regiminis et eius ordinem. — Capitulum de
ordine regiminis secundum querelas Domini Nostri — Non est   20
dubium, quod iste tractatus pervenit ad dominum meum tempore
frigoris, et propter hoc providit servus in forma regiminis, qua debet /   R198a
regi in frigido aere, sperans servus quod si dominus noster continu-
averit hoc regimen, deveniet ad pristinam sanitatem cito cum auxilio
. dei. Et quia servus ignorat consuetudinem domini mei tempore sani-   25
153r   tatis eius, utrum semel cibetur in die vel mane / et sero. Idcirco ordi-
nabit regimen secundum ambos modos. Dico ergo, quoniam oportet,
quod semper surgat a somno cum ortu solis vel parum ante, et tunc
sumat de prae / dicto sirupo ydromel sive mellicrato duas uncias vel   V15c
tres et expectet una hora, postea equitet et non cesset equitare paula-   30

---

1 et animae dillatationem H   et juvat ambas superfluitates expellere nobili juvamento V
2 praedecessore V   3 zuccario V; zucaro H   4 egiptii HV   admodum V   5 proiciat H
6 egipto HV   8 eandem (pro hanc) H   aliis (pro eis)V   omni die continue V   10 eius
om. H   in una vice H; qualibet om. H   11 allij H   12 diminutione V   14 Nam V
zucharum H   partem obtineat V   15 vinum est V   16 de hoc vino H   17 non aliud nisi V
18 Et om. H   quod om. V   19 ante memoriam eius et eius ordinem V   Capitulum . . .
Nostri om. V   20 On H   22 Et V   qua diebus debet V   24 pervenit V   25 eius sanitatis H   26 vel sero V   ordinavit V   28 semper om. V   a sompno H; a lecto V
in ortu solis vel ante parum V   29 accipiat de syrupo H; praedicto om. H   sive mellicrato
om. H   duas om. V   30 hora om. V

1 tim et suaviter et gradatim hoc faciendo, donec perveniat ad motum
velocem valde, ut membra sua calefiant et alteretur anhelitus, et tunc
descendat de equo et quiescat, donec nihil percipiatur tactu corporis
et anhelitus alterationis a labore inductae. Postea vero cibetur cum
5 aliquo praedictorum ferculorum. Deinde accipiat aliquid de fructibus
constrictivis, quos iam diximus, vel aliqua grana festucarum aut pas-
sularum aut modicum dulcedinis siccae vel modicum mellis rosati,
de quocumque illorum voluerit. Postea vero sedeat / discubito et 153v
apodiatus, donec dormiat; tunc sonator sonet cordas elevata voce et
10 acuto cantu; deinde deponat vocem per ordinem et gradatim et
mollificet cordas, donec profundetur in somnum, et tunc desinat a
percussione dordarum. Nam dixerunt medici et philosophi, quod hoc
modo somnus inductus, scilicet percussione cordarum, quaequidem
somnum provocant, facit animam acquirere bonos mores et dilatat
15 eam valde et facit ipsam bene regere corpus. Et excitatus a somno
H198d exerceat / tunc residuo diei in his, quae sibi placuerit, scilicet aut
studere in libris aut esse cum quocumque eligitur, quodquidem melius
et convenientius est, scilicet tractare et sedere cum aliquo, quem dilexerit, vel etiam aliquo negotio pietatis et misericordiae exercere vel in
20 aliquo dilectabilium et sensus lenitatis. Haec enim omnia dilatant
animam et delent ex ipsa malam cogitationem. Quod si usus fuerit,
postea sumere de cibo in sero, sumat circa libram vel tres uncias de
V15d praedicto vino cum decem drachmis / apuae rosatae et duas drachmas / linguae bovis et sumat de hoc paulatim usque in sero et expec- 154r
25 tet quasi media hora, donec exeat vinum de stomacho. Et tunc cibetur
secundum consuetudinem aliquo uno ferculorum praedictorum, / et
accedens pulsator inpediat ipsum suis cantibus et sonis duabus horis
post cibum. Tunc deponat cordas et subtiliet et debilitet cordarum
tactus, quousque dormiat, sicut fecerat in principio diei et temperet

2 et (pro ut) V   anelitus, tunc   3 ab equo H   nichil V   in tactu H   4 anelitus H
inductus V   5 dictorum V   6 quas V   8 discubito et om. H   9 appodiatus V   aut (pro
donec) V   10 donec (pro deinde) V   11 molificet H   mollificet] et debilitet V   11 in
sompnum H; in sompno V   11/12 a percusione H   12 phylosophi V   13 sompnus HV
percusione H   14 sompnum HV   acquirere animam H   15 a sompno H; excitato in
sompno V   16 in (pro tunc) V   ea (pro in his) V   placuerit sibi H   placuerit] et in quibus
plus delecetur (!) V   videlicet H   19 etiam om. H   exercere aliquid opus pietatis et misericordiae V   20 aliqua V   23 sumere de cibo postea in sero, accipiat tunc circa quinque drachmas H   22/23 de vino temperato H   25 a stomacho H   26 sicut aliquo V   praedictorum
ferculorum H   27 cantibus a sompnis V   28 Et tunc V

vinum secundum modum praedictum; et non cesset sumere de eo 1
paulatim sonantibus cordis in cantum, donec dormiat; aut post duas
horas noctis vel tres vel quattuor iuxta quod placuerit ei sedere et non
apponat intentionem ad quantitatem vini temperati, quod sumpserit,
sicut diximus; sed non dormiat. Et etiam si non sumeret de ipso 5
154v ducentas drachmas vel / trecentas drachmas aut aliquid plus tempore
hiemis, esset / utique bonum et humectaret corpus. Quod si consue- R198b
verit nihil cibi comedere cum ipso vino, comedat aliqua grana festucarum assatarum cum succo limonis vel sale. Aut sumat aliquid de corticibus citri conditis cum zuccaro aut de granis mirtae assatis aut 10
de coriandro assato, quod melius est. Quod si consueverit aliquid
cibi sumere cum ipso vino, melius quod poterit sumere est de pullis in
spico assatis, qui cibati et nutriti fuerunt cum his, quae iam praediximus sicut cum farina ordei et lacte et ficubus siccis et granis tritici.
Nec aliquis putet, quoniam comedere post cibum cortices citri condi- 15
tas cum zuccaro calefacit complexionem. Nam cotrices huius ficubus
temperatae sunt inter caliditatem et frigiditatem et sunt medicina
cordialis et ideo secure accipiat de eis post comestionem. Altero
autem die in hora excitationis a somno ducat hoc idem regimen nec
154v finis mutet aliquid / de eo, quamdiu aer duraverit frigidus, et post resur- 20
rectionem / a somno assiduet illud regimen, quod praefiguravimus. V16a
Quod si perceperit / sitim, erit sirupus secaniabin de rosis melior H198b
quam sirupus ydromellis. Quod si aliquid cruditatis inventum fuerit
in ipsa urina, tunc erit melior potus secaniabin factus de passulis. Si
vero in stomacho sentiat repletionem, accipiat decem drachmas de 25
melle rosato vel de zuccaro rosato et quattuor drachmas de trifera
praedicta, et si natura eius fuerit stricta vel sicca, subtrahat de vino,
quod bibit in nocte et diminuat comestionem in sero. Quod si consueverit comedere in sero, comedat id, quod lenificat naturam in mane et
non laboret illo die. Et nos quidem iam determinavimus in capitulo 30

---

1 praedictum modum V   2 sanantibus H   3 vel tres noctis V   eas sodare V   4 ponas V
5 si (pro sed) V   si sumpserit ex eo V   6 in tempore H   7 yemis HV   8 nichil V   9 le-
monis H   salse V   10 factis et conditis V   11 est melius quod H   consueverit forte H
tibi V   12 in ipso H   sumere de pullis est assatis in veru V   13 fuerint H   iam om. V
cum om. V   15 folia citri post cibum V   16 zucharo H   calefaciunt V   17 sunt temperati V   17/18 febris cordialis V   18 Altera V   19 sompno HV   hoc idem hoc V   20 donec
(pro quamdiu) V   Et V   surectionem H   21 sompno HV   obsiduet V   22 quod si V
secaniabim V   syrupus V   24 secaniabim V   facti F   pasulis H   25 senteat V   replec-
tionem H   26 mellis rosati V   zucharo H   26 Et accipiat tres drachmas de trifera V
28 dimittat H   29 naturam linificet H   30 in illo die   iam om. H

1 tertio huius tractatus et in praecedenti capitulo omnia, cum quibus
debebat leniri natura, et medicus, qui affuerit tunc ibi, dirigat ad ea,
quae facienda sunt. In die vero, quo voluerit introire balneum, bibat
vinum in primo, modo praedicto, et minuat de fortitudine laboris et
5 eius tempus abbreviet et ingrediatur balneum in fine laboris, et in exitu
a balneo accipiat de medicina facta ex granis granatorum et zuccaro et
specibus sicut gariofolis et mace. Et accipiat sirupum de rosis et saltim
cum aqua linguae bovis et vinum, quod scripsimus in capitulo tertio
illius tractatus et dormiat in fine balnei. Inquit Galenus: non videtur
10 mihi aliquid magis excellens in decoquendo, quod decoqui debet, et
in dissolvendo, quod debet dissolvi, quam sompnus post balneum.
Excitatus autem a somno cibetur cibo suo et studeat residuo diei et
residuis horarum noctis in his, quae praediximus, et cum cibus incepe-
rit in stomacho digeri, incipiat sumere de illo vino temperato paulatim
15 pulsante sonatore, donec perfundetur somnus secundum modum
praedictum, et non est comedendum in illa nocte aliquo modo. Et si
V16b consueverit comedere, retardet comestionem, do / nec surrexerit a
somno post eius exitum a balneo. Cum quidem voluerit coitum
R198c exercere, (R) / duas huic horas, videlicet aut / (E) cum digestus fuerit E155r init
20 cibus in stomacho, postquam sumpsit illam modicam quantitatem
vini ante comestionem in sero, vel infimae noctis. Et similiter dico,
quod ista actio non debet fieri, cum stomachus fuerit vacuus nec cum
fuerit plenus cibo. Similiter non potet vinum, dum cibus est in stomacho non digestus, quia vinum deponet ipsum crudum, nec dum
25 stomachus fuerit vacuus et requirit cibum, quia tunc calefacit complexionem et provocat dolorem capitis et urit humores, sed post cibi
digestionem. Et in qualibet hebdomada accipiat de illo electuario
mediocri, quod praescripsimus factum, scilicet cum lapidibus pre-
H198c tiosis et / non laboret illo die vel accipiat de illa trifera vel de quacum-
30 que aliarum descriptionum, quae positae sunt in canone medicinarum

2 liniri H   3 sint H   in marg. V: De balneo   in quo V   balneum introire V   5 abre,
viet HV   6 cum (pro ex) V   zucaro H   7 idem (pro Et) H   syrupum H   8 lingne V
10 michi V   excedens V   id, quod debet decoqui H   11 id, quod H   dissolve H   12 Et
excitatus H   autem om. H   14 bibere (pro sumere) V   15 sompnus om. V   16 in om. H
modo om. H   17 oportuerit (pro consueverit) V   surexerit H   18 quidem om. V   20 sumpserit H   21 communiter H   22 actio ista V   est vacuus V   23 cibi V   cum (pro dum) H
25 est vacuus V   faciet complexionem calidam V   26 capitis dolorem V   hurit H; adhurit V
sed . . . digestionem om. V   28 preciosis   30 discriptionum H   medicamentorum V

de musco. Nec consulo sumere electuarium, in quo sit castoreum 1
155v aliquo / modo, sed subtrahat castoreum in omnibus medicinis musci,
quas recepturus est dominus meus. Hoc totum est regimen domini
mei tempore, quo aer est frigidus. Tempore vero aestatis non surgat
a somno nisi post unam horam diei et accipiat de sirupo rosato et 5
passulis et sirupum, quem praediximus in quarto capitulo illius tractatus. Et laboret in frigore aeris et cibetur cum cibariis declinantibus ad
frigiditatem et dormiat ad sonum cordarum sicut iam dictum est. Et
non accipiat de illo sirupo temperato nisi modicum et non restet in
nocte vigilans et minuat coitum ab eo, quod consuetum in tempore 10
frigoris et accipiat diamuscum praedictum loco acceptionis iacut
iacinti mediocris praedictae. Quod si voluerit bibere parum de vino,
sit in fine diei, donec accipiat de eo modicam quantitatem et dormiat
in principio noctis aut in fine / secundae horae ipsius. Et si sumpserit V16c
156r de medicina iacut iacinti, / bonum est. Et sit cervisia, quam sumpserit 15
post balneum facta cum tamarindis et zuccaro et musco et modico
camphorae. Et leniatur natura, si necesse fuerit cum infusione reubarbari et tamarindorum, ut dictum est in capitulo tertio illius tractatus,
et similiter sirupum, quem praediximus. Quod si caliditas excederet,
accipiat penitus farinam de ordeo paratam omni die, cum surgit a 20
·somno ante laborem per unam horam loco praedictorum siruporum,
vel accipiat illud in lecto et dormiat super loco, quod stomachus
requirat ex cibo vel ex vino. Et modus eius, quod iuxta id, quod exigit
dominus noster, sic est: Accipiat de ordeo excorticato distante sex
mensibus a messe quadraginta drachmas seminis sahatrag contriti, 25
seminis endiviae parum contusi et linguae bovis an quattuor drachmas,
seminis papaveris acahecay parum contusi duas drachmas, sandali
156v albi contusi drachmam unam, spicae unius drachmae quartam, / flo-
rum anethi dimidiam drachmam, olei olivarum / boni occidentalis R198d
vel orientalis citrini coloris et clari et mundi a sapore amaro tres 30

3 quas recepimus pro domino meo V   4 mei incipere (pro tempore) V   extiterit (pro est) H
5 syrupo H   de (pro et) passulis H   6 syrupum H   istius V   7 exerceat V   cum om. V
8 praedictum H   Et om. V   9 accipiet H   syrupo H   stet V   10 consuevit H   11 dya-
muscum V   11/12 locam confectionis iacutorum et lapidum mediocrium praedictorum V
13 sic (pro sit) V   accepit V   ex eo H   15 iacutorum V; iacinti om. V   erit bonum H
16 zucharo H   18 tamarindis H   19/20 excederet penitus accipiat farinam V   20 paratum H
in surrectione (pro surgit) H   22 eo loco eius H   23 vel om. V   illud (pro id) V   exigat H
24 sex mensibus post eius spatium mesis H   25 X (pro XL) drachmas V   sacatas V; in marg.
H: fumaterrae   26 lingne V   acahecay: suprascr. albi H   29 aneti HV

1 drachmas, ponatur haec omnia similiter in olla et apponatur de aqua
mille drachmae, quantitas carbonum ponatur super ignem et buliant
usque ad medietatem, tunc ponantur super ipsam sex drachmae aceti
vini et perficiat eius decoctionem, donec deveniat ad quartam partem et
5 appareat eius color rubens, tunc coletur et ponatur in colatura illa
H198d dimidiam drachmam / salis et sumat illud solum absque vino semel
et sorbeat postea unam sorbitionem sirupi limonum. Et oportet
dominum nostrum considerare illud frequenter et placeat ei considerare, quoniam contradicit humori melancolico valde et rectificat hu-
10 mores acutos et eorum ustiones aufert et ingrossat vapores ascendentes
ad cor et ad cerebrum et prohibet eorum ascensum et calefacit cere-
V16d brum mediocriter et emendat omnia acciden / tia, de quibus dominus
noster conqueritur. Nam Hippocrates dicit / in omni laude ex com- E finis
moditatibus ipsius farris ordeacei, quoniam inducat, quod debet, cum
15 debet. Et non obliviscatur dominus noster eius assiduationis toto
tempore aestatis nisi natura fuerit stiptica vel stomachus acetosus vel
inflatio sub hypochondriis, quia tunc non decet domino uti eo. Et
notum est apud servum, quod bonitate intellectus domini nostri et eius
imaginationis ordinata potens est se regere modo debito ex praece-
20 denti tractatu et his capitulis et maxime, cum habuerit aliquem, qui
modificet et rectificet ipsum in arte. Et novit deus et ipse sit testis
idoneus, quia maior est voluntas servi exercere servitium domini
mei personaliter et sermone et persona quam propria pecunia et cala-
mo, sed malitia suae radicalis complexionis et eius debilitas naturalis
25 compositionis et tempore iuventutis quanto magis in senectute diviser-
unt inte ipsum et maiorem et nobiliorem convenientiam, quae possit
esse scilicet exercere et studere servitium domini nostri. Deus autem,
qui est laudabilis super omnibus rebus et negotiis in mundo generaliter
et specialiter repertis in quolibet individuo secundum eius providen-
30 tiam, quae sequitur eius sapientiam, cuius ordinem nequit homo

2 drachmae] et super ignen. ponatur cacabum V   3 usque om. H   ponatur H   octo V
5 aparebit H   coloror H   eius (pro illa) V   7 deinde (pro postea) V   sorbitionem
unam V   syrupi H   istud H   8 placeat ipsum continuare H   9 considerare] illud [quo-
niam V   melanconico H   10 vestiones V   11 ad om. V   et prohibet ... cerebrum om. V
13 ypocras V; ypo H   quae [ex V comoditatibus HV   14 ordeaci H   in (pro cum) V
15 assiduationis om. V   16 stitica H   acceptosus H   17 ypocondrijs V; ypocontrijs H
docet V   18 aput V   19 ordinata ymaginationis H   regere se H   praecedenti et tractatu V
21 fectificet et mundificet H   et novit, quod ipse   22 ydoneus HV   22 servi om. V   exerceri
officium V   23 mey H   peccunia HV   25 in tempore V   26 et nobiliorem om. V
27 studere et exercere H   28 qui in laudibus V

pertingere, sit laudatus et benedictus. Nequaquam reprehendat do- 1
minus meus servum minimum eius, quod posuimus in nostro tractatu
de usu vini et sonorum et instrumentorum, quae ambo prohibentur a
lege. Servus enim non praecepit hoc fieri, sed ostendit ea, quae ponun-
tur ab arte sua. Homines vero legum sciunt sicut sciunt medici, quo- 5
niam vinum est multorum iuvamentorum hominibus. Oportet igitur
medicum in eo, qui medicus est, narrare forman regiminis iuvantem,
sive illud in lege licitum vel illicitum. Aeger autem potest sibi eligere,
quod vult, scilicet facere aut non. Et notum est, quoniam lex mandat
quod iuvat et prohibet quod laedit in hoc saeculo. Sed differentia, 10
quae est inter mandata legalia et medicina, est haec, quoniam lex
mandans facere totum id, quod iuvaturum est in mundo, super hoc /
remunerat et prohibens facere totum / id, quod nocitivum est in V17a 199a
mundo, super hoc condemnat. Medicus vero significat, quod iuvaturum est, et prohibet, quod nocitivum est, non tamen super hoc 15
condemnat vel renumerat, sed ipsi infirmo imponit negotium modo
protestationis. Ille vero eligat, quod vult. / Et causa huius manifesta R198 finis
est, quia nocumentum et iuvamentum, quae sequuntur ex parte medicinae, apparent cito et statim fiunt nec egent remuneratione vel
poena. Mandatorum vero et legalium inhibitionum nocumenta et 20
iuvamenta non manifestantur in hoc mundo. Et ob hoc imaginatur
stultus, quod totum id, quod positum est esse nocitivum, non noceat.
Et totum id, quod positum est iuvaturum, non iuvet eo, quod non
resultat statim. Et propter hoc permittit lex pro bonis operationibus
meritum et comminnatur poena pro malis, quaequidem non mani- 25
festantur nisi in futuro saeculo. Totum hoc fuit in nostri bonum et
avantagium et suavitatem, ut miseretur nobis propter nostei igno-
rantiam et nostrae scientiae debilitatem. Hoc est, quod visum est servo
ponere inter manus domini, cuius vitam deus extendat.

---

18 dominus reprehendat V; meus om. V   servum minimum suum eius H   2 profuimus H
in tractatu nostro V   3 et sonorum om. V   4 interponunt V   5 legunt H   6 autem
(pro igitur) V   7 est medicus H   iuvamentorum V   8 et si (pro sive) V   autem om. V
9 et nobis notum V   11 quae om. V   mandata medicina H   12 mandat totum fieri, quod
est iuvaturum V   13 remuneret V   prohibet V   id om. V   nocitivum est et super V
14 condempnet V   autem (pro vero) H   15 tamen non V   super hoc om. V   17 elligat
sibi H   est manifesta H   18 quoniam (pro quia) V   iuvamentum et nocumentum V
19 nec ... poena om. V   21 modo V   22 quod ponitur est circa nocitivum V   non
possit nocere V   23 quod ponitur esse circa iuvamentum V   24 resultet V   27 misereretur
H; missetur ygnorantiam H   28 debilitatem scientiae H   29 domini nostri V
sub fine H: Explicuit omnia capitula huius tractatus et cum hoc finitus est tractatus super quo
laudeter deus excelsus.
sub fine V: Explicit consilium Raby Moysi ad yspanorum Regem de regimine sanitatis.

THE MATERIA MEDICA OF THE TREATISE
ON THE CAUSES OF SYMPTOMS

S. MARCUS

INTRODUCTION

The materia medica found in the treatise is almost entirely in line with the medical and pharmacological tradition of the Middle Ages, which itself incorporated the botanical and medical knowledge of the ancient Eastern and Mediterranean cultures from the earliest times. However, the indications for the drugs, as given by Maimonides, are not always to be found in other sources, and it is not clear whether the author at times followed some tradition which has not been handed down to us, or whether these are original observations based on his medical practice.

In addition to listing the *materia medica*—plants, animals and their products, and minerals—an attempt has been made to provide the following details: (a) the present-day terminology, or a description of the substance, or both; (b) some of the other earlier sources in which these products are mentioned; and (c) whether the substance (other than plants) is still in pharmacological use today.

The exact identification of the plants and some of the other realia mentioned in early literary sources, including those of the Middle Ages, is often rendered difficult by a lack of definition by the authors, by changes in the attribution of a particular name, or, conversely, by the existence of a number of synonyms for the same object. Even today plant taxonomy is still undergoing constant changes. Moreover, the suggested applications are often so varied and contradictory that it is difficult to decide on the exact identification of the realia. I have had no choice but to rely on the existing literature, which is mainly based on a philological approach. In general the translations and identification refer to the Arabic source of our treatise.

I have not thought it necessary to indicate all the primary and secondary sources which precede the work of Maimonides. They are mentioned to a great extent in the literature cited in the attached bibliography and in the works of the early physicians and scientists; those which are relevant here are noted above in the Medical Contents and in the Running Commentary. However, I would particularly draw attention to "Heilmittelnamen der Araber" by Steinschneider; he refers particularly to manuscript sources, most of which are still unpublished today.

In order to determine which of the old *materia medica* are still in use, I consulted the United States, British and German pharmacopoeias and other works on western pharmacognosy, especially Tschirch, who presents in his great "Handbuch der Pharmakognosie" a comprehensive account of both the natural and pharmacological properties of the *materia medica*, and their importance and use in the past; and "Hager's Handbuch der pharmazeutischen Praxis", which provides up-to-date information on the pharmaceutical usage, as well as physical and biological data. The findings shed some light on the actual state of empirical knowledge of the early physicians and on the extent to which medical practice was founded on faith and tradition without any factual basis.

In oriental cultures, this ancient knowledge has been kept alive up to the present time. Meyerhof, among others, mentions this with regard to the Mediterranean countries. Here, we cite the recently published *Hamdard* (1969), which mentions a number of drugs not mentioned in modern western pharmacopoeias, drugs that are used in the Orient to this day.

My thanks are due to D. V. Zaitschek, who checked the modern taxonomy of the plants, and who also drew my attention to a number of important pharmacological publications.

CATALOGUE OF THE MATERIA MEDICA

ABBREVIATED TITLES OF CITED BOOKS

AG	American Geology Institute, *Glossary of Geology.*
Aro	Arora, R.B., "Cardiovascular Pharmotherapeutics."
ASM	Ayalon-Shin'ar, *Arabic-Hebrew Dictionary.*
BI	*Lexikon*, Institut Bertelsmann.
BPK	Berendes, J., *Die Pharmazie bei den alten Kulturvölkern.*
CA	Adams, F., Commentary to PA: *Paulus Aegineta.*
CAS	Castellus, B., *Lexicon medicum graeco-latinum.*
CME	Clément-Mullet, M., "Minéralogie arabe."
DAF	De Biberstein Kazimirski, A., *Dictionnaire arabe-français.*
DFT	Dana, E.S. and Ford, W.E., eds., *Textbook of mineralogy.*
DHJ	*Ad-Damīrī's Ḥayāt al-Ḥayawān.*
DiB	Dioscurides, *Arzneimittellehre*, trans., Berendes.
DiD	Dioscorides, *La 'matéria médica'*, ed., Dubler.
DiS	Dioscorides, *De materia medica libri quinque*, ed., Sprengel.
DiRu	Dioscorides, *De medicinali materia . . .* ed. Ruellius.
Dozy	Dozy, R., *Supplément aux dictionnaires arabes.*
Drag	Dragendorff, G., *Die Heilpflanzen.*
Duc	Ducros, M.A.H., *Essai sur le droguier populaire arabe.*
DUS	*The Dispensatory of the U.S.A.*
DZL	Dor, M., *Zoological lexicon.*
Ergänz.bd.	*Ergänzungsband* I, II zu HHP *Hagers Handbuch der pharmazeutischen Praxis.*
EZF	Eig, A., Zohary, M., Feinbrun, N., *Analytical flora of Palestine.*
FO	Feliks, J., *Plant world of the Bible.*
GK	Galen, *Opera omnia*, ed. Kühn.
GSG	Goltz, D. *Studien zur Geschichte der Mineralnamen.*
GTL	*Grzimeks Tierleben.*
Ham	Hamdard, *Pharmacopoeia of Eastern Medicine.*
HDK	Hoppe, H.A., *Drogenkunde.*
HHP	*Hagers Handbuch der pharmazeutischen Praxis.*
HPW	Hunnius, C., *Pharmazeutisches Wörterbuch.*
HÜ	Steinschneider, M., *Die hebräischen Übersetzungen.*
IBS	Ibn al-Bayṭār, trans., Sontheimer.
IDN	Issa Bey, A. *Dictionnaire des noms des plantes.*
ISCv	Ibn Sīnā, *Canon*, trans., Sontheimer. *See* Avicenna
KAL	Al-Kindī, *Aqrābādhin*, trans., Levey.
KMU	"Die Medizin im Kitāb Mafātīḥ al'Ulūm," ed., Seidel.
KS	Kroner, H., *Der medizinische Schwanengesang des Maimonides.*
Lane	Lane, E.W., *Arabic-English Lexicon.*
LAP	Löw, I., *Aramäische Pflanzennamen.*

LFJ	Löw, I., *Die Flora der Juden.*
M	[*Maimonides'*] *Šarḥ asmā' al-ʿuqqār*, ed. and trans., Meyerhof.
MP	UNESCO. *Medicinal plants of the arid zones.*
MuA	Muwaffak, Abū Manṣūr, "Die pharmakologischen Grundsätze," trans. and ed., Achundow
MWL	*Merck's Warenlexikon für Handel, Industrie und Gewerbe*, eds., Beythien and Dressier.
NNZ	Neave, S.A. *Nomenclator zoologicus.*
PA	*Paulus Aegineta, The Seven Books of*, trans., Adams.
PF	Post, G.E. *Flora of Syria, Palestine and Sinai.*
PMG	Peters, H., *Lehrbuch der Mineralogie und Geologie.*
RPP	Remington's *Practice of Pharmacy*, eds., Martin and Cook. 1956.
RPS	Remington's *Pharmaceutical Sciences*, eds., Osol a.o. 1970.
RSA	Ruska, J., ed. and trans., *Das Steinbuch des Aristoteles.*
RSK	Ruska, J., ed. and trans., *Das Steinbuch aus der Kosmographie des . . . el-Qazwini.*
SAA	Siddiqi, H.H. and Aziz, M.A. *Avicenna's Tract on Cardiac Drugs.*
SAP	Schweinfurth, G., *Arabische Pflanzennamen.*
SAW	Siggel, A., *Arabisch-Deutsches Wörterbuch der Stoffe.*
Schm	Schmucker, W., *Die . . . materia medica im . . . Firdaus al-Ḥikma des Ṭabari.*
SCV	Steinmetz, E.F., *Codex vegetabilis.*
SHA	Steinschneider, M., *Heilmittelnamen der Araber.*
SPM	Schery, R.W., *Plants for man.*
TAR	*Tuhfat al-aḥbâb*, trans., Renaud and Colin.
THP	Tschirch, A., *Handbuch der Pharmakognosie.*
Wahr	Wahrmund, A., *Handwörterbuch der arabischen und deutschen Sprache.*
Wehr	Wehr, H., *Arabisches Wörterbuch.*
Z	Zaitschek, D.V., Personal communication.
ZFP	Zohary, M. *Flora Palaestina.*
ZTa	Hamarneh, S.K., and Sonnedecker, G., *A pharmaceutical view of . . . Abulcasis.*

*The words in parentheses appear in the Berlin and/or Munich texts,
not in the Hebrew Jerusalem manuscript*

Watermelon   *Citrullus vulgaris* Schrad.   אבטח بطّيخ

Armenian stone   אבן ארמיני حجر ارمنى

Lapis lazuli   אבן הלאזורד حجر اللازورد

Silk. Produced by *Bombyx mori* L.   אבריסם ابريسم. ראה גם משי

Prune (read: Plum) *Prunus domestica* L.   אגאץ, אפרונא أجاص. ראה גם כוך, כמתרא

Nutmeg   *Myristica fragrans* Houtt.; *M.* sp.   אגוז הוא, צ׳ל אגוז בוא جوز بواء.
ראה גם (ג׳וז בוא)

Hydromel   אדרומאלי ادرومالى

אדרציני, צ׳ל דאריציני

Jacinth   אודם ياقوت. כ׳׳י Munich (יאקות)

Stoechas   *Lavandula stoechas* L.; *L.* sp.   אוסטוכודוס اسطوخودس

Oxymel   (אוקסימל) سكنجبين. ראה סכנגבין

Iṭrīfal   אטריפל اطريفل

Spinach   *Spinacia oleracea* L.   אספנאך اسفاناخ

Opium. Secretion of *Papaver somniferum* L.   אפין افيون

Dodder of Thyme   *Cuscuta epithymum* Murr.   אפיתימון افتيمون

Prune (read: Plum) *Prunus domestica* L.   אפרונא. ראה אגאץ

Peach   *Prunus persica* Sieb et Zucc.   אפרסקים. ראה גם כוך

Citron   *Citrus medica* L.   אתרוג اترج

Basil   *Ocimum basilicum* L.   באדרוג بادروج

Balm gentle, Lemon balm, Bee balm   באדרנבויה, באדרנג׳ויה بادرنجوية, بادرنبوية,
   Melissa officinalis L.   بادرنجوية. ראה גם תרנג׳אן

Pearl   *Margarita orientalis*   בדולח لولو

Cattle   בהמות (לחם) المواش

Behen   1. *Centaurea behen* L.; *C.* sp.; 2. *Statice limonium* L.   בהמן بهمن

Fleabane, Flea seed   *Plantago psyllium* L.   בזר קטונא بزر قطونا

Balsam, Balm of Gilead, Balm of Mecca   *Commifora*   בלסאן عود البلسان
   opobalsum Engl.; et al.

Violet   *Viola odorata* L.   בנפסג بنفسج

Coral   *Corallium* sp.   בסד بسد

Purslane   *Portulaca oleracea* L.   בסד אלחתי. ראה (בקלא חמקא)

Purslane   *Portulaca oleracea* L.   (בקלא חמקא) כ׳׳יMunich. بقلة الحمقا
   ראה גם ירק השוטה, רגלה

Barberry   *Berberis vulgaris* L.   ברבאריס, ברברים برباريس
   ברכאריס, צ׳ל ברבאריס

Purslane   *Portulaca oleracea* L.   (ברדולגש) כ׳׳יBerlin. ראה (בקלא חמקא)

Apricot   *Prunus armeniaca* L.   (ברקוק) כ׳׳י Berlin. ראה משמש مشمش

Meat   *Caro*   בשר لحم

Whey   *Serum lactis*   גבינה, מי ماء الجبن

Zedoary   *Curcuma zedoaria* Rosc.; *Zingiber*   جدوار Munich (ג׳אדואר).
zerumbet (L.) Rosc.; et al.   ראה ראונד

Kid, suckling.   Young of *Capra hircus*   גדי יונק جدى رضيح

Nutmeg   *Myristica fragrans* Houtt.; *M.* sp.   جوز بواء Munich (ג׳וז בוא).
ראה אגוז הוא

Julep   גולאב جلاب

Castoreum.   Glands secretion of *Castor fiber* L.; *C.* sp.   جندبادستر ג׳נדבאדסתר
ג׳נדבאסתר, צ׳ל ג׳נדבאדסתר

Cinnamon, Cassia-bark tree (Chinese cinnamon)   دار صينى דארצ׳יני
Cinnamomum cassia Nees et Eberm.; *C.* sp.

Honey   *Mel*   عسل, ربّ דבש

Rob   ربّ דבש

Pumpkin, Field pumpkin   *Cucurbita moschata*   يقطين, قرع Munich (דלעת).
Duchesne.; et al.   ראה גם יקטין, קרא, צ׳ל קרע قرع

Greek doronicum, Leopard's Bane   *Doronicum*   درونج رومى דרונג׳ רומי
pardalianches L.; et al.

Basil, Myrtle   1. *Ocimum basilicum* L.; 2. *Myrtus communis* L.   ريحان הדס

Cardamom of Bawa, Lesser cardamom   *Elettaria*   هيل بواء. היל בוא
cardamomum (Roxb.) Maton   ראה גם קאקולא

Endive   *Cichorium endivia* L.; et al.   هندبا. ראה גם עולש הנדבא

Rose   *Rosa* sp.   ورد, וורידים

Gold   *Aurum*   ذهب זהב

(Common) Jujube   *Zizyphus jujuba* Mill.; et al.   عناب זיזב

Olive   *Olea europaea* L.   زيت זית

Emerald   زمرّد Berlin כ׳י (זמראד)

(Common) Ginger   *Zingiber officinale* Rosc.   زنجبيل זנגביל

Saffron   1. *Crocus sativus* L.; 2. *Curcuma* sp.   زعفران Munich כ׳י (זעפראן)
ראה גם כרכום, כרכומה

Zedoary, Birthwort   *Aristolochia*   djadūār תרגום מוטעה של جدوار זראונד
او حدوار ḥadūār

זרנבאד. צ׳ל זרנבאד

Zedoary root, Wild ginger, Broad-leaved finger   *Zingiber zerumbet*   זרנבאד
(L.) Rosc.; et al.

Quince   *Cydonia oblonga* Mill.; et al.   سفرجل. גם (ספרג׳ל) חבושים

Vinegar   *Acetum*   خل חומץ

Lettuce   *Lactuca sativa* L.; et al.   خس חזרת

Wheat, durum   *Triticum durum* Desf.; *T.* sp.   قمح חטה

Asphodel   *Asphodelus ramosus* L.   حنثى חתי

Suet   *Sebum*   شحم חֶלֶב

Milk   *Lac*   لبن חָלָב

Sorrel   *Rumex* sp.   حمّاض חמאץ

Bamboo manna   *Bambusa arundinacea* Willd.; *B.* sp.   طباشير טבאשיר

טברזד. ראה סוכר טברזד

Lambs.   Young of *Ovis aries*   خروف טלאים

Jacinth   ياقوت. Munich כ׳י. ראה גם אודם (יאקות)

Suckling (kid)   See *Kid*   يونق, [גדי] رضيع (جدى)

Drink, wine   *Vinum*   خمر. ראה גם משקה יין

Pumpkin   *Cucurbita pepo* L., *C.* sp.   يقطين. ראה גם קרא, צ׳ל קרע قرع יקטין

220

יקטץ צ׳ל יקטין

Blite   *Amaranthus lividus* L.   ירבוז يربوز

Purslane   *Portulaca oleracea* L.   ירק השוטה رجلة. ראה (בקלא חמקא) بقلة الحمقا

Camphor   *Cinnamomum camphora* Nees et Eberm.; et al.   כאפור كافور

Cubeb   *Piper cubeba* L.; *Cubeba officin.* Rafin.   כבאבה كبابة

Sheep   *Ovis aries*   כבשים ضأن

Pandanus palm   *Pandanus odoratissimus* L. f.   כדר كدر

כדרנגים, צ׳ל באדרנג׳ויה

Amber   *Succinum.* Fossil resin of *Pinus* sp.   כהרבא كهربا

Peach, Prune (read: Plum)   *Prunus persica* Sieb. et Zucc.; et al.   כוך خوخ.

ראה גם אפרסקים, אגאץ

Pear   *Pyrus communis* L.   כמתרא كمثرى. ראה גם אגאץ

כנדר, צ׳ל כדר

Coriander   *Coriandrum sativum* L.   כסברתא كزبرة

Saffron   1. *Crocus sativus* L.;   כרכום, כרכומה زعفران.

        2. *Curcuma* sp.   ראה גם (זעפראן)

Kashk.   Made from *Hordeum* sp.   כשך كشك

Poppy, Opium poppy   *Papaver somniferum* L.   כשכאש خشخاش

(לבונה) כ׳י Munich. ראה כדר

לומי, צ׳ל לימו

Lemon   *Citrus limon* (L.) Burm.   לימו ليمو

Oxtongue   *Borago officinalis* L.; *Anchusa* sp.   לשון השור لسان الثور

Musk   מור مسك، مسكة، مسكر

Musk.   Secretion of *Moschus moschiferus*   (מסך) כ׳י Munich. مسك

Concoctions   מושלקים مسلوق

Cucumber   *Cucumis sativus* L.   מלפפון خيار

Mastic.   Resin of *Pistacia lentiscus* L.   מצטכה مصطكة

Medicament, Electuary, Preserves   מרקחת دواء، معجون، رب

Silk.   Produced by *Bombyx mori* L.   משי ابريسم. ראה גם אבריסם

Apricot   *Prunus armeniaca* L.   משמש مشمش. ראה גם (ברקוק) כ׳י Berlin

Drink, syrup   משקה شراب. ראה גם יין

Sweetmeats   מתיקה حلواء

Water lily   *Nymphaea alba* L.   נילופר نيلوفر

Cinnamon, Malabar   *Cinnamomum citriodorum* Thwait.   סאדג׳ הנדי ساذج هندى

Folia indica.   See also: *Cinnamomum citriodorum* Thwait.

Bread made white   סולת (נקיה) حوّارى

Oxymel   סכנגבין سكنجبين

סכנומין, צ׳ל סכנגבין

Tabarzad sugar.   Sugar from *Saccharum officinarum* L.   סכר טברוד سكر طبرزد

Cinnamon   *Cinnamon* sp.   סליחה سليخة. ראה גם דאר ציני, קרפה

Senna of Mecca, Alexandrian senna   *Cassia angustifolia*   סנא מכי سنا مكة

   Vahl. *medicinalis* Bisch.; *C.* sp.

Nard   *Nardostachys jatamansi* DC.   סנבל سنبل

(ספרגאל) כ׳י Berlin. سفرجل. ראה חבושים

Quince   *Cydonia oblonga* Mill.; et al.

Crab, river   *Astacus fluviatilis* Rond.; et al.   סרטן נהרי سرطان نهرى

Endive   *Cichorium* sp.   עולש هندبا. ראה גם הנדבא

Eggplant   *Solanum melongena* L.   עכביות باذنجان

Grapes   *Vitis vinifera* L.   ענבים عنب

Ambergris, Ambra grisea. Generated in *Physeter macrocephalus*   ענבר عنبر

221

Aloe, Indian aloe tree   *Aquilaria agallocha*   עץ הנדי عود هندى.
   Roxb.; *Aloe* sp.   כ׳י Munich גם (עוד הנדי)
Brew   *Maltum hordei*   פוקעא فقاع
Fruits   פירות (פירנה) فاكهة, .pl فواكة
Pears   (פירש) כ׳י Berlin. ראה כמתרא كمثرى
Frankish musk   *Ocimum basilicum* L.; et al.   פלינג משך فلنجمشك
Pepper   1. *Piper nigrum* L., *P.* sp. 2. *Capsicum annuum* L.   פלפל فلفل
Pistachio   *Pistacia vera* L.   פסתק فستق
Currants.   Dried grapes of *Vitis vinifera* L.   צמוקים زبيب
Sandalwood   1. *Santalum album* L.; 2. *Pterocarpus santalinus* L. fil.   צנדל صندل
   צרונג, צ׳ל דרונג׳
Amomum, Java cardamom   *Amomum maximum* Roxb.; et al.   קאקולא قاقلّة
Partridge   *Ammoperdix heyi*   קורא حجل
Orache   *Atriplex hortensis* L.   קטף قطف
Snake cucumber, Cushaw   *Cucumis sativus* L.   קישואים قثّاء
Pumpkin   *Cucurbita* sp.   קרא. צ׳ל קרע قرع. ראה גם יקטין, (דלעת) يقطين
Pumpkin   *Cucurbita* sp.   קרע قرع. ראה גם יקטין, (דלעת) يقطين
Cinnamon bark   *Cinnamon cassia* Bl.   קרפה قرفة. ראה גם דאר ציני, סליחה
Rhubarb   *Rheum* sp.   ראונד راوند
Purslane   *Portulaca oleracea* L.   רגלה رجلة. ראה גם (בקלא חמקא) بقلة الحمقا
Pomegranate   *Punica granatum* L.   רמון رمون
Fumitory   *Fumaria officinalis* L.   שאהתרג׳ شاهترج
   שבה, צ׳ל שבת
Dill   *Anethum graveolens* L.   שבת شبت
Fennel   *Foeniculum vulgare* Mill.; et al.   שומר رازيانج
Oil   שמן دهن
Barley   *Hordeum vulgare* L.   שעורים شعير
Almond   *Amygdalus communis* L.; *A.* sp.; et al.   שקדים لوز
Fig   *Ficus carica* L.   תאנים تين
Dishes   תבשילין لون, .pl الوان
Turtle dove   *Streptopelia turtur, Columba turtur* L.   תורים يمام
Tamarind   *Tamarindus indica* L.   תמר הנדי تمر هندى
Apple   *Pyrus malus* L.   תפוחים تفّاح
   תרנואנג, צ׳ל תרנג׳אן ترنجان
Balm gentle, Lemon balm, Bee balm   *Melissa officinalis* L.   תרנג׳אן ترنجان
Manna   תרנג׳בין ترنجبين
Rooster   *Gallus gallus bankiva*   תרנגולין فراريج
Hen   *Gallus gallus bankiva*   תרנגולת دجاج

ALPHABETIC LIST OF ENGLISH TERMS

KEY TO SYMBOLS USED

(o)	the definition of the term
(o$_2$)	various comments
(a)	the philological basis of definition and/or physical/chemical properties
(b)	sources, selected from the literature, and/or history
(c)	pharmacological use today in both Eastern and Western medicine according to the literature cited
M.u.n.m.	modern use not mentioned in the quoted Western literature
Z	definition according to D. V. Zaitschek

MINERAL SUBSTANCES

Armenian Stone אבן ארמיני حجر ارمنی
141r 11, 12; 145v 8

(o) The identity and properties of the so-called Armenian Stone seem never to have been clear. It is not mentioned by Dioscorides, who speaks, however, of "Armenion" (Armeniacus) (liber v cap. 105, *see* GSG 113), but stresses that this substance is not a stone. *Armenion* is also mentioned in other early sources (see Pauly-Wissowa, *Realenzyklopädie*, i 1187). The misleading use of the term "Armenian Stone" for "Armenion," which occurs in the writings of Paulus Aegineta and following him in many of the editions and translations of Dioscorides, may be due to the fact that the "Armenion" appears in the list of "all the metallic stones" (liber v cap. 84-). In addition to the confusion between the nomenclature and properties of *Armenion* and Armenian Stone, they are sometimes identified with, or at least considered to re-semble, *Lapis Lazuli* (Dozy i 250; Cas 77; DiS ii 646; DiD ii 415) and *Chrysokolla*, whose properties are said to differ from those of *Armenion* only in degree. For references in the Arabic literature, see especially CME 194-8.

(a) DiS v 105, DiB 522 *Armenion*
PA iii 52 *Armeniacum*
CME 194-198
Because of the confusion of nomenclature, we are unable to specify the physical properties.
GK xix 275 L.a.: "Pro Armenio lapide, atramentum Indicum." Galen (*in:* DiRu p. 687): "Galeno lapis armenius virtutis est abstersoris cum leui quadam acrimonia, et leuissima vi astrictoria."
PA iii 221: "Used in medicine by the Ancients."
MuA p. 189
IBS i 292
GSG 147
SHA 569
Schm 229

(c) Cas 77 L.a.: Cites medical uses up to the eighteenth century.

Ham 5: "List of mineral drugs used in Unani medicine" includes: Gil-i-Armani, Hajar Armani, Boorai Armani.

(o₂) "Bolus armena (armeniaca)" is often mentioned (Cas 108). However, it is not included among the earths described by Dioscorides (περὶ γῆς liber v cap. 169 (170) — 179 (180)).

GK xii 189: mentions *B. armenia*.

DUS 1370: "The term *bolus* was formerly applied to various forms of argillaceous earth, differing in color or in place of origin . . . The most recently used of these was that called bole Armenian . . . The boles were, and perhaps some still are, used as adsorbents and protectives in various gastrointestinal inflammations".

Emerald   زمّرد (זמראד)

Ms. Berlin, **118v 4**

(a) Lane iii 1251 Emerald.

CME 64

AG 95 a bright emerald — green, variety of beryl.

DFT 580 $Be_3Al_2(SiO_3)_6$. Hexagonal; hardn. 7.5-8.; sp. gr. 2,63-2.80; 482: The "Oriental emerald" is a green corundum.

(b) RSA 98 (transl. 134)

RSK 25

SHA 949

(c) Ham 122

M.u.n.m.

Gold   ذهب זהב

145v 5

(a) AG 126, DFT 401. Au. Isometric; hardn. 2.5-3; sp. gr. 15.6 (AG 126 15.0) — 19.3 (19.33 when pure).

HHP i 595; Ergänz.bd. I 277; Ergänz.-bd. II i 770

RPS 406

GSG 255

(b) MuA 268: "Strengthens the heart."

RSA 121 (tr. 177)

SHA 852

Schm 315

(c) HHP i 595 Aurum. Medical use mentioned:

597 "Collaurin against cancer, syphilis, scrophulous illnesses, rheumatoid arthritis." See also pp. 600, 602, where the various chemical compounds and their applications are listed.

RPP 485: "Gold has been investigated extensively down through the ages with respect to possible application as a therapeutic agent for the curing of various human ills. Results have been disappointing."

DUS 1467: Between some medical uses both in the past and in the present time, no effect on heart is indicated.

Jacinth   ياقوت אודם

Ms. Munich (יאקות)

145r 10; 147r 6; 155r 13; 155v 13, 17

(a) SAW 89: "Rubin ,Saphir, Korund."

AG 66: Corundum: a mineral. Al_2O_3. Hexagonal.

AG 251: Ruby: a red variety of corundum.

DFT 481: Rhombohedral. Hardn. 9; sp. gr. 3.95-4.10.

HPW 48, CME 31: Aluminium oxydatum.

CME 30: "Chez les Arabes le mot yaqout s'applique donc à une classe de gemmes qui comprend des genres nombreux . . ."

CME 32: l'yaqout rouge.

(b) RSA 99 (tr. 135)

IBS ii 591: Cites old sources which note its good effect on the heart.

RSK 40

SHA 2033 = Rubis diamant

(c) M.u.n.m.

Lapis Lazuli   حجر اللازورد אבן הלאזורד

145v 8

(a) AG 164, 166: A mineral. $3NaAlSiO_4.Na_2S$. Isometric.

CME 191
BI 59, DFT 589 Hardn. 5-5.5; sp. gr.
2.38-2.45 (BI 59: – 2.51).
(b) RSA 107 (tr. 153)

PA iii (CA 228; 477)
SHA 1759
Schm 232
(c) M.u.n.m.

ANIMALS AND ANIMAL PRODUCTS

Ambergris   ענבר عنبر
146r 1; 147v 10
(o) In modern Hebrew, the term ‎"ענבר"
     denotes Amber. Compare also Am-
     ber כהרבא.
(a) Lane v 2168: Cites various origins as
     given in the earlier literature: "It
     issues from a source in the sea: a
     fish, marine beast, or a vegetable in
     the bottom of the sea." For a specific
     description in the medieval tradition,
     see RSK 44.
     DUS 1317 "Ambra grisea. This sub-
     stance . . . is now generally conceded
     to be produced in the intestines of the
     sperm whale (HHP i 381, HDK 1005:
     Physeter macrocephalus L.)."
     HHP Ergänz.bd. II i 472
     Ham 310, 358
(b) RSA 107 (transl. 154): Mentions
     حجر العنبري the "Ambrastein", which
     he says resembles the عنبر "Ambra".
     On the difficulties of definition and
     other problems, see RSA p. 56.
     RSK 29, 44 ditto, (44 عنبر).
     SHA 1406
     Schm 502
(c) DUS 1318: A. "was formerly regard-
     ed as a cordial and antispasmodic,
     somewhat analogous to musk, useful
     in . . . various nervous diseases."
     HHP i 381: Only formerly used as
     stimulant and aphrodisiac.
     HDK 1005: In hysteria, neurasthenia,
     nervous states, sleeplessness.
     Ham 310

Castoreum ג'נדבאסתר, ג'נדבאאדסתר جندبادستر
146r 13; 147r 2; 155r 16, 17; 155v 1
(a) M 79

Duc 225
DUS 1388 "In the beaver, *Castor
fiber* L., between the anus and external genitals of both sexes, are two
pairs of membranous follicles . . .
containing an oily, viscid, highly
odorous substance, secreted by
glands which lie externally to the
sac."
Ham 371
HHP i 870, HDK 979 cite *Castor fiber*
from Siberia and Canada (*C. f.* L.
var. *canadensis* Kuhl); THP I ii 860
cites also *C. norwegicum* and *bavari-
cum.*
HHP Ergänz.bd. II i 847
(b) DHJ I 481
     SHA 476
     THP I ii 859: Mentions many sources
     and various applications in medicine
     up to the nineteenth century.
(c) DUS 1388: "Castor was at one time
     much used as a stimulant, antispas-
     modic, also as an emmenagogue, but
     has passed out of medical use."
     HHP i 871: Antispasmodic. HDK 979:
     Also used as a nerve tonic and for
     chest diseases.
(o₂) Castor should not be confused with
     Castor oil
     RPS 798, 478: = *Oleum ricini*, derived
     from the seed of *Ricinus communis*
     L. (*Euphorbiaceae*).

Cattle בהמות (לחם) المواشى
149v 16 בשר
(a) ASM 350
     HHP i 832: Lists the main chemical
     constituents of the meat of cattle and
     other animals.

Coral   بسد בסד
145v 2; 146v 6; 147v 1

(a) Various species were used for their medicinal effects, including:
Corallium album
THP I ii 823 *Madrepora occulata* L.
HHP i 737, HDK 1000 *Oculina virginea* Less. Little used.
Corallium nigrum
THP I ii 823 *Gorgonia antipathes*.
Corallium rubrum
M 45, HHP i 737, Ergänz.bd. II i 905, HDK 985 *C. r.* Lamm.; THP i 823 *Gorgonia nobilis* Sol. Consists mainly of calcium carbonate and small quantities of magnesium, iron compounds, chitin-like substances, traces of iodine compounds.
In ancient times the biological nature of بسد (*basad*) was not clear:
RSK 9 Considered it to be a stone growing in the sea like a tree on the earth.
RSA 120 (tr. 176), M 45: Defined it as a plant. Another name for coral is مرجان *mardjan*. According to M 45, there is no unanimity as to whether بسد בסד denotes the "root" (RSK 9) or the branches (M 45) of the coral.

(b) SHA 271
Schm 125

(c) The old sources mentioned above agree as to its value in the treatment of palpitation of the heart and in dispersing melancholy and promoting hilarity.

Crab, river   سرطان نهري سرطان נהרי סרטן
145v 3; 147v 2

(a) HDK 973, THP I ii 807 *Astacus fluviatilis* Rond.
HHP Ergänz.bd. I 362 *Potamobius astacus* L. (*A.f.* Rond.)
Duc 169

(b) DHJ II i 43 سرطان
SHA 994

(c) THP I ii 807: Used from early times

and in Arab medicine. No mention of use in heart disease.
Also HDK 973 promotes bone formation; formerly used against gastric hyperacidity.

Hen   دجاج תרנגולת
148v 10; 149r 1, 7; 150r 5; 151v 3

(a) Lane iii 852: The common domestic fowl, both cock and hen.
DZL 353, GTL viii 50, 51 *Gallus gallus bankiva*
ASM 102 תרנגולת
HHP i 832: Gives the chemical analysis of chicken meat.

(b) SHA 800

(c) THP I ii 818 *Caro galli*

Honey   رب, عسل דבש
145r 3; 146r 4, 10; 147r 1; 147v 3, 13; 151v 16

(o) Only once, 151v 16, does the term "honey" refer to bee honey عسل النحل. It is prescribed as an ingredient of hydromel.
In 145r 3, "honey" is used to describe the consistency of a preparation (قوام العسل). In all other cases, the Hebrew דבש is a translation of the Arabic *robb* رب.

(a) HHP ii 146, 1341; RPP 1022, DUS 541-2: Description of the composition and consistency of honey.
THP II i 8
HHP Ergänz.bd. I 791, II ii 1332

(b) SHA 1367, THP II i 14, Schm 486

(c) THP I ii 867. Modern use DUS 542, THP II i 14.
RPP 285; DUS 542
HHP ii 153: Recipe for oxymel (simplex) and other preparations made from honey.
THP II i 14
See also the list of *Medicaments and Foods;* Rob (p. 247)

Kid, suckling   جدى رضيع (יונק) גדי
149v 16

(a) DZL 243 Young of *Capra hircus*

GTL xiii 537 *C. aegagrus hircus* Hausziege
ASM 49

(b) DHJ I 404: Explains and points out its beneficial properties.

Lambs טלאים خروف
150r 2

(a) ASM 90
DML 143, 159 Young of *Ovis aries*
GTL xiii 553 *O. ammon aries*

(b) DHJ I 673

Meat בשר لحم
140v 8; 142v 9; 148v 10; 149v 15, 16; 150r 1; 151r 12; 151v 6

(a) HPW 162, HHP i 832: List the main chemical constituents of various kinds of meat.

(b) THP I ii 817: From earliest times meat was used in the diet and for medical purposes. Mentions the use of various kinds of meat in the medicine of the past, particularly in Arabic literature.

(c) Ham 304

Milk חלב لبن
137r 4; 149r 12; 149v 4; 154v 11

(o) *Lac*

(a) RPP 936, HHP i 832, Ergänz.bd. I 741, HHP ii 39, Ergänz. bd. I 741, II ii 1288

(b) SHA 1765

(c) THP I ii 864

Musk מור مسك, مسكة, مسكر
144v 16; 146r 1; 147v 9; 146r 2 מור مسك
144v 5 دواء مسك
146v 2 מורה مسكة
155r 16; 155v 2, 12 دواء مسكر

(o) The Hebrew and Latin texts translate as מור *mur*, and "*muscus*" respectively, three terms occuring in the Arabic manuscripts: مسك, مسكة, مسكر, which denote different substances. Our identifications refer to the

Arabic terms, but an exact definition depends on the vowelization, which is lacking in our text espec. at مسكر. As to the Hebrew translation, מור is generally *Commiphora* sp. (PF i 284 *C. abyssinica* Engl.; ? *Bals. Mukul* Hook.; Arab. *murr;* Heb. *mor.* MP 70 *C.* sp.), especially in Biblical times (LFJ i 305 ff, FO p. 252, THP III ii 115). In our treatise, this meaning does not correspond to the Arabic texts and the early Latin translations. In medieval Hebrew literature מור also denotes "musk" (Moschus). (Maimonides in his *Mishne Tora*, Hilkot Berakot, 9.1 says: "Mor comes from an animal," a statement which is repeated in his other writings (Hilkot Berakot, 1.3; his commentary to Mishnayot, *Miqwa'ot*, 9.5). (See also J. Kna'ani x 3284; viii 2697, 2725). See LFJ i 310 for further sources which demonstrate the confusion about the meaning of the term. Probably this ambiguity is due to the fact that all these substances possess a strong odor.

(a) Lane viii 3020: "It is obtained from the . . . musk-deer, *Moschus moschiferus;* being found in the male animal in a vesicle near the navel and prepuce".
DAF ii 1106
LFJ i 310
Wahr ii 798
THP II ii 1157, HHP ii 183, Ergänz.-bd. I 803, II ii 1344
Z: *Misk* is Moschus only

(b) IBS ii 513

(c) THP II ii 1160
HHP ii 185
Several medical preparations made from musk, mentioned in 155r 16, 155v 12, are found in Avicenna's *Canon* (ISC v 33-35, 96).
See *Musk* also in the lists of *Medicaments and Foods* and of *Plants and Plant Products*.

Partridge كورא حجل
149v 13

(a) Lane ii 520: Cites Arabic sources referring to its physical and medicinal properties, but no mention is made of the indications given by Maimonides.
DZL 303 *Ammoperdix heyi* = Desert partridge
ASM 66

(b) DHJ I 509: Contains no direct indication regarding its action in "kindling the mind": "its flesh is of a moderate temperament, delicate, easily digested."

Pearl بدولح لولو
145v 2; 147v 1

(a) CME 16, 17 لؤلؤ la petite perle
פנינים = בדולח 17
THP I ii 881 *Margarita orientalis*
DUS 245: "Calcium carbonate occurs in nature in several different forms. Native forms include ... pearl, coral, and various shells."

(b) PA iii, (CA 473)
RSA 53 בדולח در; 96 (tr. 130).
IBS ii 446
Schm 687

(c) THP I ii 881: In the past used mainly as an ingredient of expensive prescriptions for heart conditions, particularly in medieval Arab medicine.
DUS 245: In the modern pharmacopoeia, there is no indication of use in heart diseases.
M.u.n.m.

Rooster (should read Pullet) תרנגולין فراريج
148v 11; 150v 4; 154v 9

(a) DHJ II i 557
Lane vi 2360: The young of the domestic hen
DZL 353, GTL viii 50, 51 *Gallus gallus bankiva*
DAF ii 562 poulet
Wahr ii 406 junges Huhn
ASM 267 אפרוח

Sheep כבשים ضأن
150r 1

(a) ASM 204
DZL 159 *Ovis aries*, GTL xiii 553 *O. ammon aries*

(b) HHP i 832: The chemical composition of the meat of the sheep
SHA 1245 ضأن

(c) THP I ii 818: *Caro ovile*. It is good for the digestion (Ibn Sīnā) and produces good blood (Abū Manṣūr Muwaffaq b. 'Alī al-Harawī).
M.u.n.m.

Silk אבריסם, משי ابريسم
145v 3; 147v 2

(a) Dozy i 2; SAW 11
HDK 974, HHP ii 1003, THP I ii 807, II i 504 produced by *Bombyx mori* L.
Ham 364

(b) SHA 10

(c) Ham 119-120
M.u.n.m.

Suckling kid يونק (גדי) رضيع (جدى)
149v 16; 151v 6

(a) ASM 127
See Kid, suckling גدى (יונק) جدى رضيع

Suet חֵלֶב شحم
149v 5

(a) ASM 175
HHP ii 675
Lane iv 1513
RPS 1380 Suet: "Internal fat of the abdomen of the sheep, *Ovis aries* (*Bovidae*)."
THP II i 729 *Sevum ovile;* II i 730 *S. bovinum*
HDK 1002, HHP ii 676, Ergänz.bd. II 1542 *Sebum ovile*

(b) SHA 1135
THP II i 731

(c) Uses: in ointments and cerates.
The medical use of chicken fat is only mentioned in old pharmacopoeias (THP I ii 838).

Turtle dove   تورים يمام
149v 11
(a)   ASM 432
    DZL 346, GTL viii 262 *Streptopelia*
    turtur
    THP I ii 816 *Columba turtur* L.
(c)   THP I ii 816, 818: No reference to
    "kindling the mind" in the older
    literature is found here.
    M.u.n.m.

Whey   מי גבינה ماء الجبن
141v 2; 142r 3, 9
(a)   HHP ii 55 *Serum lactis*, THP I ii 866
    Molken

HHP ii 52: Liquid residue from the
cheesemaking.
Its components: 6.5-7.5 percent dry
matter, composed of 60-70 percent
milk-sugar, protein-like stuff circa
1 percent.
(b)   DiS, DiB, liber II, cap. 76, 77. DiB
    p. 176: explains how whey is made
    and refers to its further properties.
    MuA 256
    SHA 427
(c)   THP I ii 866: In earlier times given as
    laxative.
    HPW 449: Sometimes mixed with
    drugs, and so on.

PLANTS AND PLANT PRODUCTS

Almond   שקד(ים) لوز
142r 7; 150v 12
(o)   *Amygdalus communis* L.
(a)   LAP 319
    HHP i 410, Ergänz.bd. I 205,
    Ergänz,bd. II i 490
    Drag 282,   PF i 449
    ZFP ii 21
    Two varieties:
       1. Sweet almond: var. *dulcis* Mill.
       THP II i 594, HHP i 417.
       2. Bitter almond: var. *amara* Hayne
       THP II ii 1473, HHP i 410 *Prunus*
       amygdalus Stokes
    EZF 88: *Prunus amygdalus* Stokes
(b)   SHA 1792 — 5: 1. 1794, 2. 1795
    THP II i 607, II ii 1477
    Schm 685
    Schery 407
(c)   Almond oil: Ham 306
    THP II ii 1476; HHP i 411, 417
    RPS 767, MP 77

Aloe, Indian aloe tree   עץ הנדי (עוד הנדי)
145v 7-8, 147v 4-5   عود هندى
(a)   Drag 458, M 296 = عود الطيب *Aquilaria*
    agallocha Roxb. (*Thymelaeaceae*)
    Ham 361 Ud el-juj 357 *Aloe indica*
    THP II ii 1421 *Aloe* sp.

(b)   Schm 509, 506
    THP II ii 1440
(c)   Ham 361, 357
    RSP 796
    MP 18–19, 60–61 *Aloe* sp.

Amber   כהרבא كهربا
144v 14; 145v 2; 147v 1
(o)   *Succinum*
    In the literature, there is some con-
    fusion between Amber كهربا and
    Ambergris عنبر, see below. In modern
    Arabic كهربا is "electricity."
(a)   THP I ii 859 Medici Florentini:
    Ambra citrina = succinum = Elek-
    tron = Charabe.
    Tschirch, A. et al. "Ueber den
    Bernstein". *Helvetica Chimica Acta*
    6 (1923): 214–225: "Harz von
    Pinus succinifera (sowie *P. baltica,*
    silvatica und *cembrifolia*)."
    HHP ii 805
    DFT 776 Hardn. 2–2.5; sp. gr. 1.096.
    "Amber and similar fossil resins are of
    vegetable origin, altered by fossili-
    zation. Amber was known to the
    ancients under the name ἤλεκτρον."
    DUS 1317: "A fossil or semifossil
    resin . . . from Pinites (HPW 665,

HHP ii 805, HDK 691 *Pinus succini-fera.*)"
BI 59 $C_{10}H_{16}O$. Amorph.
PMG 239
(b) M 199
RSK 33
HÜ 701 note 321: Cites the Hebrew translation of Avicenna's *De viribus cordis*, which describes its properties in connection with those of the jacinth.
SHA 1747
Schm 657
(c) RPP 1018: Amber, succinum a fossil which contains succinic acid, and a volatile oil (Oil of Amber), which is stimulant and antispasmodic, or rubefacient, when applied externally.
DUS 1317: "Amber was held in high estimation by the ancients as a medicine, but at present is never so used. The pharmaceutical uses of amber are discussed by Walden (*Pharm. Ztg.*, 1936, **81**, 321)."
HPW 665 In popular medicine: antispasmodic.

Amomum   קאקולא قاقلّة
145v 10
(o) Z *Amomum maximum* Roxb.
(a) M 325: Points out the difficulty of exact definition.
Drag 145: *Amomum granum Paradisi* L. (*Zingiberaceae*) = Kâkulah.
THP II ii 1071, HHP i 823, Ergänz.bd. I 387, II i 836 *Elettaria cardamomum* White et Maton.
Duc 81: *Elettaria major* Smith.
KAL 313, 314: *Amomum* sp.
(b) SHA 1520
Schm 561

Apple   תפוח(ים) تفّاح
137v 10; 139r 4; 140r 7; 145r 2; 147r 1; 147v 12; 148r 2
(o) *Pyrus (Pirus) malus* L. (*Rosaceae*).
(a) Drag 274–5
PF i 454

(b) SHA 387
Schm 169

Apricot   משמש (ברקוק) مشمش
139v 11; 140r 13
(o) *Prunus armeniaca* L. (*Rosaceae*).
(a) LAP 105, M 233, PF i 453
Drag 283: Arab. Mischmisch = Berkuk.
HHP ii 516
(b) SHA 1877
Schm 729

Asphodel   חתי حنثى
146v 6
(o) The Arabic sources differ in the spelling of the name of this plant. (Kroner edition): Huntington gives حبثى, Pocock קתי, Paris חני. The meaning of the Latin translation "spodium" is also not clear. The correct reading may well be حنثى *Asphodelus ramosus* L. (*Liliaceae*).
(a) M 395
LAP 233, p. 291
HHP Ergänz.bd. I 276
(b) KAL 230
Drag 115–6: Ibn al Baiṭār, and in Morocco today known as *Chanta* (*Ablalutz Chanta*) = A.r.L.

Balm gentle; Lemon balm; Bee balm
I באדרנג'ויה بادرنجوية
באדרנבויה بادرنبوية
כדרנגים بادرنجبوية
148r 5; 148r 13
(o) *Melissa officinalis* L. (*Labiatae*)
THP II ii 879; HHP ii 156; Ergänz.bd. I 792, II ii 1334
(a) Drag 579, M 40 in Egypt = ترنجان
Ham 406: *Nepeta hindostana* Ham.
(b) SHA 226
THP II ii 883
Schm 94
(c) Ham 406, 473, Aro 447

II תרנג'אן ترنجان
137v 12
(a) Drag 579, M 40, PF ii 345
KS 91

(b) SHA 384
Schm 165=94

Balsam; Balm of Gilead; בלסאן
Balm of Mecca عود البلسان
146v 12
(o) *Commiphora opobalsamum* Engl.
(a) Drag 368: Also *Balsamodendron gilea-
dense* Kth., *Amyris gileadensis* L.
(*Burseraceae*).
PF i 284
For the discussion of the identification
of *Commifora* see THP III ii 1115
HHP Ergänz.bd. I 286
Ham 363
(b) SHA 319
THP III ii 1128
Schm 139
(b,c) Schweinfurt, G., "Ueber Balsam und
Myrrhe." *Berichte der pharmaceu-
tischen Gesellschaft*, 5. 10. 1893.
THP III ii 1127
HHP Ergänz.bd. I 286
RPS 777, MP 70 *Commiphora* sp.

Bamboo Manna طباشير טבאשיר
147r 1; 147v 6
(o) *Bambusa arundinacea* Willd. (*Gramineae*).
(a) M 171, Drag 89: The silicate con-
cretions on the nodes of the cane,
which are frequently used in medicine,
are known as *Tabashīr*.
THP II i 132: "1. Tabaschir findet sich
an der Oberfläche einiger indischer
Bambusarten, bes. *Bambusa stricta*
Roxb. = σάκχαρον des Dioscorides:
"Honig des Zuckerrohrs."
2. "Tabaschir kommt im Inneren der
Bambushalme vor."
Duc 148
Ham 363
PF ii 795 *Bambusa* sp.
(b) KS 96
C. C. Hosseus. "Die Beziehungen
zwischen Tabaschir, Bambus-Manna
oder Bambus-Zucker und dem Σάκχα-
ρον der Griechen". *In:* Beihefte zum
Botan. Centralblatt 30 (1912): Abt. II.

SHA 1263
Schm 464
(c) Ham 363

Barberry برباريسى ברברים, ברכארים
צ״ל ברבאריס
137r 13; 137v 4
(o) *Berberis vulgaris* L. (*Berberidaceae*)
(a) Drag 232 *Berberis* sp.
PF i 29
HHP i 666; Ergänz.bd. I 307
(b) SHA 249
Schm 71
(c) HHP i 667

Barley شعير (ים) שעורה
**138r 3, 9; 138v 12; 149r 12; 149v 3;
154v 10; 156r 7, 13**
(o) *Hordeum vulgare* L. (*Gramineae*).
(a) Drag 88
PF ii 793
THP II i 197
HHP i 1438
(b) SHA 1151
Schm 431

Basil, sweet بادروج באדרוג
145v 6 *see* ראה פלינג משק
(o) *Ocimum basilicum* L. (*Labiatae*).
(a) Drag 586–7, *O.b.* L. = Raihan
(el-melk, Farandsch musk.)
PF ii 328
HHP ii 257, Ergänz.bd. I 839
Duc 112 = ريحان كبيرة
M 48
Ham 407
(b) SHA 227
HHP ii 258
Schm 95
(c) MP 83 *Ocimum* sp.

Basil; Myrtle ريحان הדס
137v 11
(o) The meaning of ريحان is not precisely defined. This term designates a
plant (according to ASM 136 all
plants) of sweet odor, esp. *Ocimum
basilicum* L. (Lane iii 1181) and also

231

Myrtus communis L., (Wahr i 814, SHA 914, ASM 136, KS 91). The Hebrew translator chooses the last meaning.

(a) 1. Duc 112 *Ocimum basilicum* L. (*Labiatae*) = ريحان also sweet basil بادروج .
PF ii 328

2. Duc 4 *Myrtus communis* L. (*Myrtaceae*) = ريحان in Egypt, Arabia and Yemen; هدس in Southern Arabia.
HHP ii 199, Ergänz.bd. I 807, II ii 1347
PF i 468
ZFP ii 371
Ham 405

(b) SHA 914
Schm 334 → 332
HHP ii 200

(c) Ham 405
MP 83 *Ocimum* sp.
78 *M. communis* L.

Behen   בהמן بهمن
145v 7; 147v 5

(o) *Centaurea behen* L. (*Compositae*).

(a) PF ii 113 *C.b.*L.
1. white: M 50, Duc 47, EZF 288
Drag 686 *Centaurea cerinthifolia* Sibt. (*C. behen* Lam., *Serratula beh.* DC.)
HHP i 886
2. red: Duc 154 *Statice limonium* L. (*Plumbaginaceae*). This has also been suggested, with some reservations, by Drag 515, LFJ iii 68, Z.
PF ii 413 *S.l.* L. = *Limonium vulgare* Mill.

(b) Schm 152
Ham 372: Does not distinguish between white and red behen.

(c) Ham 372

Blite   ירבוז يربوز
150v 15

(a) EZF 28, Z: *Amaranthus lividus* L. (*Amaranthaceae*).
Drag 200, M 53 *Albersia blitum* Kth. = *Amaranthus blitum* L. = *A.l.*L.

ZFP i 186 *Amaranthus gracilis* Desf. = *A.l.*L. = *Albersia blitum*.

(b) SHA 2039

Camphor   כאפור كافور
146r 1; 146v 14; 156r 3

(o) Z *Cinnamomum camphora* Nees et Eberm. (*Camphora offic.* Nees) (*Lauraceae*).

(a) Drag 240
THP II ii 1110
PF ii 482
RPS 773
HHP i 768, ii 1314; Ergänz.bd. I 356, II i 800
Duc 66 = *Curcuma zerumbet* Rosc., Camphore des gateaux.
Ham 367 *Camphora officinarum* Bauh.
HHP Ergänz.bd. II i 800

(b) SHA 1632
THP II ii 1132
Schm 610

(c) THP II ii 1132
HHP i 770
RPS 774

Cardamom of Bawa;   היל בוא هيل بواء
Lesser cardamom
145v 9

(o) *Elettaria cardamomum* (Roxb.) Mat. (*Zingiberaceae*)

(a) Drag 145, M 116
THP II ii 1071
HHP i 823, Ergänz.bd. II i 836
Duc 80 *E. c.* Mat. = قاقلة صغيرة Petit Cardamome
Ham 382

(b) SHA 2004
THP II ii 1082
Schm 781 also هال

(c) Ham 382

Cinnamon; Cassia bark (Chinese cinnamon)

(o) In the older Arabic literature, there is no clear distinction between دار صيني, قرفة, سليخة
Z All these terms have been used for *Cinnamomum cassia* and also for *C. zeylanicum* Nees. According to

TAR 112, 291, M 95, Z, the Arabs did not know the C.z.N. Nevertheless the verbal meaning of دار صينى is "Bark of China."
The plant: HHP i 869, 1016, 1019, Ergänz. bd. I 453, II ii 846.
The bark: HHP i 1019; ii 1318; Ergänz.bd. I 453, II i 879
ZFP ii 32 – Cassia sp.

Cinnamon   סליכה سليخة
145v 9
(a) Drag 239 Cinnamomum sp. (Lauraceae). M 95 C. cassia Bl.
Duc 127 C. c. Blum. قسيا = قرفة.
TAR 112 = κάσσια = C. aromaticum Nees. = Laurus cassia L.
(b) SHA 1046
Schm 399

Cinnamon, bark of   קרפה قرفة
151r 1
(a) ASM 289, TAR 112 قرفة: bark, espec. bark of Cinnamon
Drag 239 Cinnamomum sp. "Bei Ibn el Baiţâr = Dâr Sînî, Salicha et al. (Kirfat, Kurfa, d.h. Rinde ueberhaupt). Welche Rinde aber gemeint ist..., ist meistens nicht festzustellen."
Drag 239, THP II ii 1261, M 95 Cinnamomum cassia Bl. (Cinn. aromaticum Nees, Cassia cinn. Fr. Nees)
Duc 181 C. zeylanicum Breyn. = دار
صينى = قرفة سيلان = قرفة الطيب
127 C. cassia Blum. = قرفة = قسيا.
RPS 1337
(b) SHA 1550
THP II ii 1270
Schm 570
(c) Schery 258, 262 C. cassia
THP II ii 1270

Cinnamon, Cassia bark (Chinese   דארציני
cinnamon)   دار صينى
142v 10; 145v 9
(a) Z Cinnamomum cassia Nees et Eberm. (Lauraceae)
THP II ii 1261 C. c. (Nees von Esenbeck) Blume; HHP Ergänz.bd. II i 879

M 95 C. zeylanicum Nees: Not known to Greeks and Arabs.
C. aromaticum Nees: Dār şīnī = bois de Chine.
TAR 112, 291 = κίνναμον. C.a. Nees = Laurus cassia L.: la cannelle de Chine
KS 115
(b) SHA 792
THP II ii 1270
Schm 292
Duc 181 Cinnamomum zeylanicum Breyn: = قرفة

Cinnamon, Malabar   סאדג׳ הנדי سادج هندى
see
Folia indica

Citron   אתרוג اترج
145r 4; 146v 12; 147r 12; 150v 10; 154v 6, 12, 14
(o) Citrus medica L. (Rutaceae)
(a) Drag 359, FO 70, PF i 277
Drag 359 اترج = ليمون
THP II ii 843, 873
HHP i 1032, 1036
M 1 C.m. L. lageniformis Roem.
Ham 374
(b) SHA 17
THP II ii 851
Schm 4
(c) Ham 374

Coriander   כסברתא كزبرة
139r 9,11; 139v 2; 144v 14; 150v 6; 154v 6
(o) Coriandrum sativum L. (Umbelliferae).
(a) THP II ii 835
HHP i 1106, Ergänz.bd. I 491
PF i 533
ZFP ii 401
(b) SHA 1687
THP II ii 840
Schm 635
(c) HHP i 1107

Cubeb   כבאבה كبابة
145b 10
(o) Piper cubeba L. (Piperaceae)

233

(a) Lane vii 2583: "A certain medicine of China."
Drag 157 = *Cubeba officin.* Rafin.
Duc 195 *P.c.*L. كبابة هندى = كبابة صغيرة.
THP III i 182
HHP i 1126, Ergänz. bd. I 501, II i 911
M 194

(b) SHA 1637
THP III i 192
Schm 616

(c) HHP i 1128
THP III i 192

Cucumber خيار מלפפון
136v 10
(o) *Cucumis sativus* L. (*Curcurbitaceae*)
(a) PF i 480 Hebr. *Ḳishū'im*
HHP i 1130
(b) SHA 782
Schm 286
(c) Ham 378

Currants زبيب צמוקים
150v 12; 153r 14; 155v 6
(o) Dried grapes of *Vitis vinifera* L. (*Vitaceae*): Passulae
(a) Dozy i 578: Dried currants, also all dried fruit, except dates.
Wine or cold drink made of dried currants.
Lane iii 1208: Dried grapes; or raisins; and also dried figs.
THP II i 39
PF i 283
HHP ii 969
(b) SHA 930
THP II i 42
Schm 339
(c) THP II i 42

Dill شبت שבה
should read שבת צ״ל
156v 1
(o) *Anethum graveolens* L. (*Umbelliferae*)
(a) Drag 498, M 363
THP II ii 1105
PF i 554
HHP i 439, Ergänz.bd. I 215, II i 529
ZFP ii 433

(b) SHA 1119
THP II ii 1106
Schm 420
(c) HHP i 440, Ergänz.bd. II i 530

Dodder of Thyme افتيمون אפיתימון
145v 11; 146v 3; 142r 1, 2, 7
(o) *Cuscuta epithymum* Murr. (*Convolvulaceae*)
(a) KS 93
‗ PF ii 214
HHP Ergänz.bd. I 505 *C.* sp.
(b) SHA 134
Schm 54

Doronicum, Greek; דרונג׳ רומי
Leopard's bane درونج رومى
145v 14; 147v 5 (צרונג)
(o) Z *Doronicum pardalianches* L. or *Doronicum caucasicum* Bieb.
(a) Drag 683 *Doronicum scorpioides* Lam. (*Compositae*)
PF ii 67 *D.c.*M.B.
HHP Ergänz. bd. II i 754 *Doronicum* sp., et al.: *Arnica montana*
KAL 267 *D.p.*L.
M 81: Possesses the same properties as جدوار.
(b) SHA 814
Schm 300

Eggplant باذنجان עכביות
140v 8
(a) LAP 142, Drag 591 *Solanum melanogena* (PF ii 258, Z: *melongena*) L. (*Solanaceae*).
(b) SHA 228 Melangia; Aubergine.
Schm 96

Endive عولش هندبا הנדבא, עולש
135v 3; 136r 11; 145v 15; 147v 15; 148r 1; 156r 16
(o) M 114: General name for some *Chicoraceae*, esp. *Cichorium endivia* L. (*Compositae*), et al .
(a) LAP 195
THP II i 203, HHP i 1007, Ergänz.bd. I 449, II i 875

PF ii 124
Drag 694 also *C. intybus* L.
Ham 372 *C.i.L.*
EZF 292 *C. pumilum* Jacq. עולש מצוי
(b) SHA 2001
THP II i 205
Schm 789
(c) THP II i 205
Ham 372

Fennel שומר رازيانج
150v 7
(o) *Foeniculum vulgare* Mill. (*Umbelliferae*)
(a) Drag 491–2, M 351
THP II ii 1185 *Pimpinella anisum* L.,
1194 *Foeniculum capillaceum* Gilibert.
Duc 136 *F. dulce* Bauh.
PF i 544
HHP i 1303, Ergänz.bd. I 599, II ii 1033
Ham 386 Badiyan
(b) SHA 855
THP II ii 1192, 1203
Schm 318
(c) Ham 386
THP II ii 1192, 1203
HHP i 1305
MP 38

Fig تين תאנים
139v 14; 149r 13; 149v 3; 154v 11
(o) *Ficus carica* L. (*Moraceae*)
(a) Drag 172
THP II i 24
PF ii 515
HHP i 826
ZFP i 37
(b) SHA 405
THP II i 34
Schm 180
(c) THP II i 33
HHP i 828

Fleabane, Flea seed بزر قطلونا בזר קטונא
137b 13
(o) *Plantago psyllium* L. (*Plantaginaceae*)
(a) Drag 618, M 52, Duc 36
THP II i 337
PF ii 422
HHP ii 484, Ergänz.bd. I 956, II ii 1442

(b) SHA 266 also قطلونا
Schm 121
(c) HHP ii 484, Ergänz.bd. II ii 1443
MP 47–48

Folia indica, סאדג׳ הנדי
Malabar cinnamon سادج هندى
146r 2
(o) *Cinnamomum citriodorum* Thwait. (*Lauraceae*).
(a) Drag 240: Known as Sâdadsch by the Muslims.
HHP i 1019 *Cortex Cinnamomi (ceylanici)*: *Cinnamomum* sp.: Ceylon-(Java-, Malabar-) zimt
LAP 209 *Laurus malabathrum*
(b) SHA 974
Schm 361

Frankish musk فلنجمشك פלינג משך
145v 6
(a) Drag 586, LFJ ii 78, Ham 407 *Ocimum basilicum* L. (*Labiatae*)
HHP ii 258, Ergänz.bd. I 839
Drag 587, M 47 *O. pilosum* Willd.
M 47 also *Calamintha* sp.
KS 97
(b) SHA 1489, 1460
Schm 543 — 529 فرنجمشك

Fumitory شاهترج שאהתרג׳
136v 4; 146v 4; 156r 15
(o) *Fumaria officinalis* L. (*Fumariaceae*)
(a) M 358
PF i 44
HHP i 1322, Ergänz.bd. I 606
Ham 387
(b) SHA 1107
Schm 416
(c) Ham 387
HHP i 1323

Ginger زنجبيل זנגביל
146v 13
(o) *Zingiber officinale* Rosc. (*Zingiberaceae*)
(a) THP II ii 1044
زنجبيل برّة = عرق الطيب Duc 117
HHP ii 994, Ergänz.bd. I 1182, II ii 2050

(b) SHA 952
     THP II ii 1056
     Schm 355
(c) THP II ii 1056
     HHP ii 995
     Ham 416

Grapes   ענבים عنب
139v 13

(o) *Vitis vinifera* L. (*Vitaceae*)
(a) PF i 283
     HHP ii 969, Ergänz.bd. I 1174
(b) SHA 1400
     Schm 500

Jujube   זיוב عناب
135v 4, 9

(o) Z *Zizyphus jujuba* Mill. (*Rhamnaceae*).
(a) Drag 410–1, M 291 *Zizyphus sativa*
     Gaertn.
     PF i 289 *Ziziphus officinarum* Medik.
     HHP ii 996
     EZF 147 *Zizyphus* sp. שיזף
(b) SHA 1399
     Schm 499
(c) MP 71

Lemon   לימו, לומי ليمو
150v 4, 10; 151r 9; 151v 2, 5; 154v 5;
156v 11

(o) *Citrus limon* (L.) Burm. (*Rutaceae*).
(a) Drag 359 *Citrus limonum* Risso. "Bei
     Alidrîsi scheint eine Var. als Limûah
     vorzukommen, während die Araber
     sonst die Zitrone Atrog' (Utrudsch)
     und Limun nennen."
     THP II i 541, 543; II ii 843, 873
     PF i 277
     HHP i 1024, 1036, Ergänz.bd. II i 881:
     Citrus medica L. subsp. *limonum*
     (Risso) Hooker f.; et al.
(b) IBS ii 452 ليمواو ليمون Limo oder
     Limon
     THP II ii 851
     SHA 1802

Lettuce   חזרת خسّ
136v 10; 147r 13

(o) *Lactuca sativa* L. (*Compositae*)

(a) Drag 691
     THP III ii 831—
     PF ii 146
     HHP ii 65, Ergänz.bd. I 746, II ii 1295
     Ham 396 Bazr-ul-Khas *L. scariola* L.
(b) SHA 746
     Schm 270
(c) Ham 396
     THP III ii 835
(o₂) In modern Hebrew the term חזרת
     designates
     Z: *Armoracia lapathifolia* Gilib. (*Cruci-
     ferae*)
     Drag 253 *Cochlearia armoracia* L.

Manna   תרנג'בין ترنجبين
(o) According to Maimonides (M 166, 386:
     "Tarangubīn: c'est ce qu'on appelle
     manne (*mann*) et on l'appelle aussi
     rizq (provision)"), these three names
     are synonymous. Since ancient times
     manna has been considered as "dew
     of the heaven" (Tarangubīn: M 166,
     386, TAR 259, IBS i 207, KHM 5
     "*mann-es-samā*'). In accordance with
     this conception 1) رزق "*rizk*" means
     a gift, especially of God; the support,
     substinence, sustenance . . . which
     God sends; something good or
     excellent; a daily allowance of food,
     etc. (Lane iii 1076, Wahr i 755);
     2) مَنّ "*mann*," as a verb "donner,
     faire une grace", as a noun "manne",
     but also "certain insecte qui est
     nuisible aux arbres" (Dozy ii 616,
     KHM 6, LFJ iii 403).
     It seems, that "tarandjubīn"[1] primarily
     designates the sweet matter from
     Persia[2], which possesses peculiar
     properties (MP 73). Later it was used
     to express, *pars pro toto*, also other
     species. In the Sinai peninsula, the
     Beduins attach the term *mann* (the

---

1) Vullers, I.A. *Lexicon persico-latinum etymologicum*. Bonnae, 1855. i 440.
   Steingass, F. *A comprehensive Persian-English
   dictionary*. London [1892]. p. 297; IBS i 207.
2) Murray, J.A.H. *A New English Dictionary*.
   Oxford, 1908. vi 118–129.

Biblical manna) to the sweet products which exude from the *Tamarix* sp., *Haloxylon* ("very close" or synonymous to *Hammada* (ZFP I text volume, p. 164)), *Artemisia* and other plants.

(a) As to the origin of manna itself, several sources and ways of production are known. These are
 1) the sugary exudation of certain plants;
 2) the sugary secretion of certain insects after sucking the sap of particular plants;
 3) the thallus of the lichen *Lecanora esculenta* Ev. (*Sphaerothallia* esc.).

For recent investigations see

Kaiser, Alfred. "Der heutige Stand der Mannafrage". *Mitteil. d. Thurgauischen Naturforschenden Gesellschaft.* 1924, Heft 25: 1—59.

Bodenheimer, Fritz Simon und Theodor, Oskar. *Ergebnisse der Sinai — Expedition* 1927. Leipzig, 1929.

Bodenheimer, Fritz Simon. "The Manna of Sinai". *The Biblical Archaeologist* 10(1947): 2—6.

Danin, Avino'am. "The manna that our fathers ate". *Teva' wa-arez* 11 (1969): 222—224 [In Hebrew].

See also THP II i 131. Other kinds of Manna: p. 103.

HHP ii 138; Ergänz.bd. I 789—: Other sources of Manna.

DUC 223

KS 91

(b) SHA 385

(c) MP 72—73
 Kaiser, 1924: Medicinal use in Sinai not known.

Mastic מצטכה مصطكة
142v 11; 145v 9; 151r 1

(o) Resin of *Pistacia lentiscus* L. (*Anacardiaceae*)

(a) THP III ii 1138, PF i 286, HHP ii 141, 478, Ergänz.bd. I 789, II ii 1331
 Duc 220 *P.l.L.* var. *chia* DC.

EZF 145 *P.l.L.* אלת המסטיק
ZFP ii 299
Ham 312, 411

(b) THP III ii 1141, SHA 1879
 Schm 730: According to 'Alī ibn Rabban aṭ-Ṭabarī it is synonymous with كية (Schm 664).

(c) THP III ii 1141, Ham 312, 411

Musk מור مسك, مسكر

It is not sure whether مسك *musk*, resp. مسكر *muskir* refer in our treatise to plants, and therefore their definition does not seem to be relevant to our contest. In any case, there exist some plants bearing this name:
Dozy ii 592: مسك several plants.
Duc no. 149: مسكر الحوت *Anamirta cocculus* Wight et Arn. (*Menispermaceae*): "boisson qui enivre le poisson".

See Musk also in the lists of *Animal and Animal Products* and *Medicaments and Foods* resp.

Nard סנבל سنبل
142v 11; 146r 2; 151r 2; 156r 18

(a) Dozy i 690: Common name of several plants.
 Lane ii 1440: A certain plant of sweet odor.
 THP III ii 1106 "Sumbul ist ein arabischer Sammelbegriff und bedeutet soviel wie Kolben oder Ähre (ear or spike). Speziell die indische Narde wird so bezeichnet."
 M 265 "Sunbul est le nom arabe de toutes sortes de nards".
 HHP ii 817, Ergänz.bd. I 1091, II ii 1707: *Euryangium sumbul* Kauffmann, et al.
 LAP 316
 Drag 645 In Turkestan Sumbul et tib. M 265 *Nardostachys jatamansi* DC. (*Valerianaceae*).
 Aro 422–434

(b) SHA 1067
 Schm 403

(c) THP III ii 1106, Ham 406, Aro 422–434

Nutmeg   אגוז הוא جوز بواء
should read ג״ל אגוז בוא

146v 12

(o) *Myristica fragrans* Houtt. (*Myristicaceae*).

(a) Ham 404
THP II i 665, HHP ii 188, Ergänz.bd. I 805, II ii 1346
Drag 218 *M.f.* Houtt., also *M. moschata* Thbg., *M. offic.* L., *M. aromatica* L. = Muscatnuss.
Duc 68, M 71 = جوز الطيب.

(b) SHA 481 = جوز الطيب
THP II i 686
Schm 209

(c) Ham 404
THP II i 685

Olive   زيت זית

156v 1

(o) *Olea europaea* L. (*Oleaceae*)

(a) THP II i 608
PF ii 182
HHP ii 258

(b) SHA 967
THP II i 623
Schm 359, 360

(c) Olive oil THP II i 622, HHP ii 260, Ham 307
MP 80

Opium   افيون אפיון

146r 12, 16

(o) Z: Medicinal opium is a preparation of the dried milky secretion of the plant *Papaver somniferum* L., which merges after incisions are made in the unripe pericarp.
Papaver somniferum L. (*Papaveraceae*)

(a) Lane i 70: "From the Greek ὄπιον. The milk (or juice) of the black Egyptian خشخاش, (or poppy, or *Papaver somniferum*)." He cites medieval sources which refer to biological properties and medicinal applications.
THP II i 563, III i 592, HHP ii 309, 385, 1349, Ergänz.bd. I 871, II ii 1375

THP III i 593 "Zur Opiumgewinnung wird fast überall *Papaver somniferum* var. γ *album* DC. . . . gebaut."
M 35
PF i 36
RPS 1121—
MP 43–44 *P.s.L.* or its variety *album* DeCandolle. Records the chemical components and some medical effects of opium.

(b) SHA 136
THP II i 569, III i 644
Schm 60

(c) THP III i 643
Ham 408
HHP ii 321, 386
RPS 1121
MP 44
See also Poppy, Opium poppy خشخاش
כשכאש (p. 240)

Orache   قطف קטף

136v 12

(o) *Atriplex hortensis* L. (*Chenopodiaceae*)

(a) M 150 = خمّاض. "*Qataf* est un nom arabe qui désigne plutôt des espèces d'arroche (par exemple *Atriplex hortensis* L.)."
SHA 1586
Schm 583

Oxtongue   لسان الثور לשון השור

133r 10; 133v 8, 9, 14; 134v 6; 145v 4; 147r 11, 15; 154r 1

(o) *Borago officinalis* L. (*Boraginaceae*)

(a) LAP 182, Drag 561, M 211
M 211 also *Anchusa italica* Retz. (= Drag 562: Buglossa, i.e. lingua bovis; EZF 201 *Anchusa* sp. לשון הפר).
PF ii 224 *B. officinalis* L.
HHP Ergänz.bd. I 212 *Anchusa officinalis* L., 319 *Borago officinalis* L.; II i 289
SHA 1781

(b) Schm 675

Pandanus palm   (رتّ, خشب) כדר كدر, כאדי

147v 3, 4

(o) In the Arabic manuscripts, the name of

this plant is spelled in two forms: Huntington, Pocock: كادر, Paris: כאדי. It is not clear whether this is an error of the scribes (if so, the correct form should be כאדי كادى: Pandanus palm), or whether these are synonymous names for the same plant (see Drag. 74). Ibn-al-Bayṭār distinguishes between كاذى *Kādhi*: the tree *Pandanus odoratissimus* and its wood, and (according to Eltamimi) الكدر *Alkadr* (Elkader): the wine made from it. Our Jerusalem text transcribes כדר. In Ms. Munich 280 (135r 16) it is translated as כנדר (עסים the sap = דבש) and לבונה (the tree). These versions are possibly based on a misreading of the sources, or on other, lost text traditions (לבان = كندر = χόνδρος = כנדר): Frankincense; Lane vii 2633). In any case, the distinction in the Arabic language between the wood and its products is expressed in the Munich Hebrew manuscripts.

Pandanus odoratissimus L. f. (*Pandanaceae*)

(a) Dozy ii 434, KAL 320
Drag 74 *P.o.*L. f.: "In Arabien Kadi, Kadar, Kadsu genannt."
IBS ii 337 كاذى *P.o.*; 338: The wine of this plant is known by the name الكدر: *Elkader* (according to Eltamimi).
KS 99 —

(b) SHA 1630

(c) Ham 310 mentions *Aqua Pandanus odoratissimus* عرق كيورة "obtained by distilling fresh *P.o.* flowers with water". Perhaps this aqua may be identical with the "Robb of *P.o.*"

Peach, Prune (read Plum)   כוך خوخ
see also ראה גם אפרסקים, אפרסקיה, אגאץ
140v 1; 141v 5; 142v 8; *see also* 150v 16
(o) *Prunus persica* Sieb. et Zucc.
(a) also *Persica vulg.* DC. *Amygdalus persica* Lam. (*Rosaceae*).

LAP 105 1: in Egypt: *A.p.* Lam., peach.
2: اجاص = *prunum, malum Persicum.*
In Egypt: *choch*: Pfirsich, *barkuk*: Pflaume.
PF i 452 *P. domestica* L.
HHP ii 516, Ergänz.bd. I 972
KS 93
(b) SHA 777
Schm 283

Pear   כמתרא כّّثרى
see also ראה גם אגאץ
139v 12; 140r 7
(o) *Pyrus (Pirus) communis* L. (*Rosaceae*)
(a) Lane vii 2630 (in Egypt)
Dozy ii 487
Drag 276, M 187: اجاص = (idjāṣ) in Maghrib (Maimonides: M ;87), in Syria (M 187, IDN 151: عامة الشوام) and Yemen (M 187, LAP 153, Lane ibid).
PF i 453: *najāṣ*.
(b) DiS I 167, p. i 151, ii 417 "Pyrorum multa sunt genera".
PA i 130; CA i 134
IBS ii 388
SHA 1725
THP II ii 791
Schm 648

Pepper   פלפל فلفل
146b 13
(a) Dozy ii 279
1. Drag 154, IDN 141,2 Black pepper: *Piper nigrum* L. (*P. aromaticum* Lam.) (*Piperaceae*): فلفل اسود (*fulful aswad*)
THP III i 168
HHP ii 465, 470
2. Drag 595, IDN 39, PF ii 259, Z: *Capsicum annuum* L. (*Solanaceae*); SCV no. 240 *C.a.* var. *longum* L. et al. =*fulful (filfil) ahmar; f. rūmy.*
THP III ii 867 *C.a.L.; C.sp.*
HHP i 793
(b) 1. DiS II 188 (189) p. i 298, ii 475 *Piper* sp.
PA iii 294
IBS ii 261
KAL 311

239

SHA 1483
Schm 538
THP III ii 877

(c) 1. THP III i 180
HHP ii 469
2. THP III ii 876
HHP i 795

Pistachio פסתק فستق
151r 7; 153r 14; 154v 4

(o) *Pistacia vera* L. (*Anacardiaceae*).
(a) Drag 395, M 301
PF i 286
HHP ii 478
(b) SHA 1465
Schm 530

Pomegranate רמון رمون
139r 5; 139v 14; 147v 13

(o) *Punica granatum* L. (*Punicaceae*)
(a). PF i 469
HHP i 1382, Ergänz.bd. I 626, II i 1059
(b) SHA 896
THP III i 335
Schm 329
(c) THP III i 334
MP 78–9

Poppy, Opium poppy כשכאש خشخاش
138r 4; 138v 13; 156r 17

(o) *Papaver somniferum* L. (*Papaveraceae*)
(a) SAP 34, Duc 55, Ham 408 *P.s.*L.
THP III i 593 "Zur Opiumgewinnung
wird fast überall *Papaver somniferum*
var. γ *album DC. . .* gebaut."
PF i 36
HHP ii 309, 385, Ergänz.bd. I 920, II
ii 1375
Drag 249 = "Mohnpflanze, mit weis-
sem Samen."
THP II i 563 *Semen* and *oleum papave-
ris.*
M 401 "*ḥašḥāš* est aujourd'hui le nom
générique arabe de tous les pavots".
See also Duc 55.
MP 43–44 *P.s.*L. or its variety *album*
DeCandolle.

(b) SHA 749
THP III i 644
Schm 273
(c) HHP ii 321, 386, 387
THP III i 643
MP 44
Ham 408
See also Opium افيون אפיון (p. 238).

Prune, (read Plum) اجاص אגאץ, אפרונא
see also Pear, Peach ראה גם כמתרא, כוך
135v 4, 9; 138r 9; 138v 14;
150v 15 [והוא שקורין אותו אנשי אר]ץ]
יש [ראל] (اهل الشام) כוך)

(o) There are various meanings of the
Arabic name اجاص, according to
the geographical area and the historical period (see among others Lane
i 24, Dozy i 10, KS 93). This lack of
exact nomenclature is also reflected
in the different translations into
Hebrew. Here the identification as
plum has been chosen in conformance with the term used in Egypt,
where Maimonides composed his
treatise.
(o) *Prunus domestica* L. (*Rosaceae*)
(a) Lane i 24: Lists many medicinal
applications.
THP II i 57
PF i 452 *P.d.* var.*juliana* L.
HHP ii 515, Ergänz.bd. I 973
KS 92, 93
(b) SHA 22
Schm 7
(c) M.u.n.m.

Pumpkin יקטין, קרא, (דלעת)
(o) In the botanical historical literature
there is great confusion about the
identification of these plant names
in both Hebrew and Arabic. It seems
that in the Arabic tradition قرع
קרע is generally synonymous with
יקטין يقطين (TAR 116: *al-qar'* =
al-yakṭīn, M 332). As to דלעת
(in MS. Munich 280, 135r 13 for
قرع), it is not clear whether the

Arabic term دلّاع denotes a species of *Cucurbita*. Probably, it is an erroneous translation of قرع *Ḳar'*.

يقطين يقطين (יקטץ)
138r 4, 7; 138v 13; 150v 4
(o) *Cucurbita pepo.* L. (*Cucurbitaceae*)
(a) M 332 *C.p.*L.; also *C. maxima* Duch., *Lagenaria vulgaris* Ser. In Egypt denotes قرع *Cucurbita* sp., *Lagenaria* sp.
Drag 652
HHP i 1130, Ergänz.bd. I 502
KS 92

קרא قرع
147r 13 *should be* ק'ל קרע
(o) *Cucurbita pepo* L. (*Cucurbitaceae*)
(a) LAP 297 קרא *Cucurbita pepo* L.
Maim. دلّاع
Drag 652 *C.p.*L.
M 332 p. ٣٦ [36] Maimonides:
"قرع هو الدباء ويعرفة عامة مصر باليقطين"
"Qar' ... le peuple d'Égypte le connaît sous le nom *d'el-yaḳṭīn*."
PF i 483 *C. moschata* Duch.: *Ḳar'* in South
EZF 253 *Cucurbita* sp.
(b) SHA 818 دلّاع *Citrulus* 1548 قرع
Schm 569
(c) HHP i 1131

(דלעת) قرع
MS. Munich 280 **135r 13**
(corresponding to **147r 13**)
(a) Z: ?*Cucurbita moschata* Duch.
LAP 297 דלעת = קרא *Cucurbita pepo* L. Maim. دلّاع
Drag 652
M 98 دلّاع: *Citrullus vulgaris* Schrad. et sp. In Arabic: certain varieties of بطّيخ
EZF 253 *Cucurbita* sp.
(b) SHA 818 دلّاع *Citrul* 1548 قرع

Purslane רגלה, ירק השוטה, בסד אלחתי, (בקלא אלחמקא) رجلة, بقلة الحمقا
رجلة **136v 11; 139v 6; 151r 4**
بقلة الحمقا **146v 6; 147r 15**
(o) *Portulaca oleracea* L. (*Portulaceae*)

(a) Lane i 236, 646 = رجلة (Garden Purslane)
Drag 205
PF i 220
HHP Ergänz.bd. I 968
ZFP i 78
(b) SHA 304
Schm 33

Quince חבושים, (ספרג'אל) سفرجل
139r 4; 139v 12; 140r 7; 147v 13
(o) Z *Cydonia oblonga* Mill. (*Rosaceae*)
(a) Drag 274, THP II i 328, Duc 26 *Cydonia vulgaris* Pers., *Pirus cydonia* L.
PF i 454 *C. oblonga* Mill.
EZF 85 *C. oblonga* Mill. חבוש מוארך, THP II i 328 *C.o.*Mill. = Birnquitte
HHP i 1154, Ergänz.bd. I 506, II i 926
(b) SHA 1017
THP II i 336
Schm 383
(c) THP II i 335
HHP i 1154

Rhubarb راوند ראונד
136r 10; 136v 1; 141v 2; 156r 4
(o) *Rheum* sp. (*Polygonaceae*)
(a) Drag 189–190
THP II ii 1366
LAP 126, Duc 107 *Rheum palmatum* L.
108 *Rheum rhaponticum* L.
EZF 16 *Rheum* רבס
HHP ii 563, Ergänz.bd. I 991, II ii 1485
(b) SHA 861
THP II ii 1386
Schm 321
(c) THP II ii 1386
HHP ii 568

Rose ورد ורד
135r 1; 135r 6; 134v 19; 144v 13; 145v 17; 146v 5; 147v 7; 148r 3,6,7, 10; 151r 6, 16; 151v 2; 152r 12; 153r 15; 154r 1; 155v 5
(o) *Rosa* sp. (*Rosaceae*)
(a) PF i 458
ZFP ii 15–
THP II ii 791
HHP ii 581, Ergänz. bd. I 998

(b) SHA 2012
THP II ii 812
Schm 797

(c) THP II ii 812

Saffron زعفران (זעפראן) ,כרכום
145v 9; 146v 2 כרכומה, ;זעפראנה **147v 8;**
151v 8, 9

(o) Both כרכום, זעפראן and زعفران may
serve as synonyms for *Crocus sativus*
L. and for *Curcuma longa* L. (M 135,
205).

(a) 1 *Crocus sativus* L. (*Iridaceae*). Z:
זעפראן, زعفران
Drag 139, THP II ii 1453, M 135,
SPM 243, 256, FO 249, Ham 377
PF ii 583 *C*. sp.
HHP i 1120, ii 1320, Ergänz.bd. I 498,
II i 910

2. Z: *Curcuma domestica* Valet.: כרכום
LAP 162, THP III ii 909, M 205,
FO 249: root of *Curcuma longa* L.
(*Zingiberaceae*)
HHP i 1152, Ergänz.bd. I 505, II i 926
Duc 209 root of *Curcuma* rond =
زعفران الهند

(b) SHA 941
THP II ii 1466, III ii 914
Schm 349 *Crocus sativus* L. var. *culta
autumnalis*

(c) Ham 308, 377
1. HHP i 1123, 1153
THP II ii 1463
THP III ii 914 "*Curcuma* spielt als
Arzneidroge keine Rolle. Es ist
Farbdroge und dient . . . zur Ver-
fälschung anderer Drogen . . ."

Sandalwood صندل צונדל
134v 20; 135v 3; 136v 8; 146v 6;
156r 18

(a) 1. Drag 183, Ham 412, Duc 146 *Santalum
album* L. (*Santalaceae*): صندل ابيض
s. white
THP II ii 950
HHP ii 636, Ergänz.bd. I 1013, II ii
1499
2. Drag 327, Duc 147, THP II ii 962, III

ii 924 *Pterocarpus santalinus* L. fil.
(*Leguminosae*) (red) صندل احمر s. red
HHP ii 636, Ergänz.bd. I 1013, II ii
1499

(b) SHA 1237
THP II ii 961
Schm 461

(c) Ham 412
THP II ii 960
HHP ii 639

Senna of Mecca, Alexandrian סנא מכי
senna سنا مكة
146v 5

(a) Drag 302 *Cassia angustifolia* Vahl.
medicinalis Bisch., et var.
LFJ ii 407–
ZFP ii 33 *Cassia senna* L., *Senna alex-
andrina* Gars., et al.
PF i 440 *C. obovata* Collad.
THP II ii 1408 *C. angustifolia* V.
HHP ii 691, Ergänz.bd. I 1036, II ii
1555
LAP 329, EZF 126 *Cassia acutifolia*
Del. (*Leguminosae*)
M 267 i.e., also *C. obovata* Collad.
MP 26–, 74
Ham 370

(b) SHA 1065
THP II ii 1419

(c) Ham 370
THP II ii 1419
HHP ii 694, 695
MP 27, 74

Snake cucumber, cushaw قثاء (ים)קישוא
136v 11; 145v 16; 147r 14

(o) *Cucumis sativus* L. (*Cucurbitaceae*)

(a) LAP 278, Drag 650, Duc 176 *C.s.*
LAP 278 also *Cucumis chate* L.:
Maim. קשות (see LAP p. 436).
HHP i 1130
PF i 480 *C.s.*L.
PF i 483 *Cucurbita italica* Tod. Arab.:
kusa
EZF 252–3 *C.s.*L. קשוא הגנה

(b) SHA 1528
Schm 562

(c) Ham 378

Sorrel   חמאץ حمّاض
137v 10

(o) The Hebrew transliteration does not take into account the diacritical point over the last letter of the Arabic word ض, which changes the pronounciation, to ḍ. The Hebrew צ *Z* refers to the root of the Hebrew word חמץ (= sour, acid).

(a) Drag 191 *Rumex* sp. (*Polygonaceae*). *?R. acetosa* L. and *?R. obtusifolius* L.
LAP 125 *R. acetosa* L.
HHP ii 591, Ergänz.bd. I 1002, II ii 1490
M 150
PF i 253 *Oxalis* sp.
Duc 90 *Oxalis acetosella* L.
See also THP II ii 1395: Rumexdrogen

(b) SHA 696
Schm 251

Spinach   אספנאך اسفاناخ
136v 11; 150v 14

(o) *Spinacia oleracea* L. (*Chenopodiaceae*)
(a) PF ii 432
(b) SHA 74
Schm 28

Stoechas, Lavender   אוסטוכודוס اسطوخودس
145v 11

(o) *Lavandula stoechas* L. (*Labiatae*)
(a) THP II ii 831 *Lavandula dentata* L., *Lavandula officinalis* Chaix., and *L.* sp., see p. 823—
PF ii 328
HHP ii 78, 74 Ergänz.bd. I 750
MP 82
(b) SHA 72
THP II ii 831
Schm 28
(c) THP II ii 830

Sugar, Tabarzad   סכר טברזד
see Tabarzad sugar

Tabarzad sugar   סכר טברזד سكر طبرزد
148r 4, 3

(o) Sugar from *Saccharum officinarum* L. (*Gramineae*), cane sugar.

(a) Lane v 1822 "Sugar-candy... or excellent sugar."
Drag 78
M 289: "signifie le sucre solide et dure"
PF ii 704
KAL 284: According to Levey, "Ṭabarzad sugar is crystalline and is considered to be the finest."
KS 96
(b) SHA 1030
Schm 391

Tamarind   תמר הנדי تمر هندى
135v 4; 142v 8; 151r 3; 156r 2, 4

(o) *Tamarindus indica* L. (*Leguminosae*)
(a) Drag 299, THP II i 528, M 381, Duc 52
HHP ii 843, Ergänz.bd. I 1115, II ii 1829
(b) SHA 392 b
THP II i 540
Schm 173
(c) THP II i 539
HHP ii 845

Violet   בנפסג بنفسج
136v 5

(o) *Viola odorata* L. (*Violaceae*)
(a) PF i 150 *V.* sp.
ZFP ii 334
HHP ii 966, Ergänz.bd. I 1170, II ii 1965
(b) SHA 342
Schm 151
(c) HHP ii 967

Water lily   נילופר نيلوفر
143r 7, 141v 9

(o) *Nymphaea alba* L. (*Nymphaeaceae*)
(a) PF i 30 *N.* sp.
ZFP i 217
Drag 211, EZF 46
HHP Ergänz,bd. I 839, II ii 1352
M 252 *N. lotus* L. var. *alba*
Duc 38 *N. lotus* L.
(b) SHA 1982
Schm 779 *N.* sp.

Watermelon   أبطيخ بطّيخ
139v 13; 140r 12; 141v 5; 147r 13

(o) *Citrullus vulgaris* Schrad. (*Cucurbitaceae*)

(a) M 54
PF i 480

(b) PA i 128: (The summer fruits) "upon the whole, all this class of fruits are of a cold and humid nature, supply little nourishment, and that of a bad quality."
PA i 129 (CA): "Melons (in general) are said by Averrhoes to be of a cold nature, juicy, detergent, and diuretic."
MuA 345
SHA 294
Schm 131

(c) Ham 374

Wheat, Durum   قمح حطה
148v 2; 149v 1; 145v 11

(o) *Triticum durum* Desf. (*Gramineae*)

(a) Lane vii 2561
Drag 87, THP II i 184 *T. vulgare* Vill.
PF ii 783
EZF 331 *Triticum* sp.

(b) THP II i 188, 157
Schm 595 *T. sativum*

(c) THP II i 188

Zedoary root, Wild ginger,   زرنباد זרנבאד
Broad-leaved ginger
145v 13; 147v 5

(o) *Zingiber zerumbet* (L.) Rosc. (*Zingiberaceae*)

(a) Drag 142
HHP ii 994, Ergänz.bd. I 1182, II ii 2049 *Zingiber officinale* Rosc.
M 145 "la drogue est la racine de *Zingiber Zerumbet* Rosc."
THP II ii 1058 *Curcuma zedoaria* Rosc.
Duc 66 *Curcuma zerumbet* Rosc.

(b) SHA 937

THP II ii 1062
Schm 345 *Amomum zerumbeth*

(c) HHP ii 995

145v 12   זראונד

(o) The Hebrew translation זראונד in our text of the جدوار، حدوار in the Arabic sources is not exact and probably erroneous. See also MSS. Munich 134b 7 גאדואר, by mistake גאדואד, and the Latin translations: *zedoarae* (*zedoariae*). In Hebrew these two terms designate different plants.
See Zedoary (ג'אדואר). It seems that this confusion was widespread (see Drag 188).

(a) זראונד: LAP 225 *Aristolochia*
Drag 187, M 133 *Aristolochia longa* L. (= *A. sempervirens* L.) and *A. rotunda* L. (= *A. sempervirens* and *A. pallida* Wiild.) (*Aristolochiaceae*)
ZFP i 48 *A. sempervirens* L.
HHP Ergänz.bd. I 253, II i 753 *Aristolochia* sp.
Drag 188: "Mitunter wird unter dem Namen Zirawand etwas ganz anderes verkauft."
Duc 114 *A. rotunda*

(b) SHA 933   زراوند
Schm 189

Zedoary   جدوار (ג'אדואר)
see ראה זראונד *MSS.* Munich כ"י
MS. M 280, 134v 7 גאדואר; MS. M 87, 127v 21

(a) Drag 143, THP II ii 1058 *Curcuma zedoaria* Rosc. (*Amomum zedoaria* L., *Curcuma zerumbet* Roxb.) (*Zingiberaceae*). *See* Zedoary root זרנבאד.
HHP ii 974, Ergänz.bd. I 1177 *C.z.R.*
M 81

(b) SHA 431
THP II ii 1062
Schm 189

(c) HHP ii 975

MEDICAMENTS AND FOODS

Bread made white   سولت (נקיה) حَوّارى
148v 2
(a) Lane ii 666: White or whitened; the best and purest flour; applied also to bread.
(b) SHA 713 pain de fine farine.

Brew   פוקעא فقّاع
156r 1
(a) Lane vi 2428: A certain beverage.
    HHP ii 122 *Maltum hordei*
    KS 83 Gerstengetränk.
(b) SHA 1477
    Schm 535: Belongs to the اشربة syrups.

Concoctions   מושלקים مسلاّق
142v 13
(a) Lane iv 1411: "What is cooked with hot water, especially of herbs, or leguminous plants."

Dishes   תבשילין pl. لون, الوان
**150r 15, 17; 150v 8; 151r 9, 12, 14;
151v 1; 154r 4; 155v 7**
(a) Lane viii 3015: Sorts, or species, of viands.
    ASM 339

Drink, syrup   משקה شراب
See also Wine, Syrup — יין גם ראה

Exhilarating drink   "משקה משמח שלאק
should read התלמיד" ציל של אבן התלמיד
137v 7, 10
(a) DUS 1177: "Syrups are concentrated aqueous solutions containing sugar, either with or without the addition of medicating or flavouring ingredients . . . it receives its specific name from the (medicinal) substance or substances added."
    HHP Ergänz.bd. I 970 *Potiones*
    Ham 169

Electuary   מרקחת معجون
See Medicament

Fruits   פירות (פירנה) pl. فاكهة, فواكة
140r 3, 5, 9, 10; 140v 5
(a) ASM 276: Fruits, sweets.

Hydromel   אדרומאלי ادرومالى
151v 15; 152r 1
(a) Dozy i 14
    HHP ii 153 *Hydromel simplex*
(b) PA i 178
    ISC v 117 The description differs from that given in *De causis accidentium*.
(c) HHP ii 153: Modern recipe for hydromel (simplex).

Itrifal   אטריפל اطريفل
155r 14
There exist various kinds of *Iṭrīfal*. In our treatise no specification is mentioned.
(a) Dozy i 28
    ZTa 70 "The tryphera (= I.) is a . . . confection in dough form, its basic constituents are the three medicinally-famous myrobolans."
    40: The tenth treatise of the *Kitāb al-Tasrīf liman 'Ajiza 'an al-Tālīf* includes a discussion on Iṭrīfal.
(b) ISC v 26, 85, 98: I. magnum; 85: I. parvum.
    KMU 60, 61
    Schm 48
(c) Ham 65-72, 314

Julep   גולאב جلاب
147v 15; 148r 5
(a) ZTa 135: "A sweetened mixture or drink, made from various medicinal preparations that were usually kept in the form of a dough."
    BPK ii 149: Lists five kinds of julep from the *Antidotarium of Mesue*,

245

according to their floral ingredients.
They are simple syrups.
HHP Ergänz.bd. I 970

(b) IBS ii 689-698: Treats of the distillation
of the julep.
ISC v 113, 114
Schm 200

(c) M.u.n.m.

Kashk (Barley kashk)   كشك כשך
156r 7

(a) ASM 316: A food made of wheat and
sour milk (in modern Arabic).
HHP i 1438 *Hordeum* sp.
KMU 25, 28: "Wheat or barley,
pounded in a mortar till the separation of the hull"; also gruel.

(c) DUS 1480: "Barley (*Hordeum vulgare*
L.) in the form of the decoction,
popularly known as barley water,
affords a mucilaginous drink much
employed from the time of Hippocrates to the present ... it seems to
prevent the formation of large milk
curds by its protective colloidal
character."

Medicament, Electuary,   מרקחת
Preserves   دواء, معجون, ربّ
144v 5; 145r 9; 151r 6; 155r 13

(a) In Arabic, there is a distinction between
1) دواء medicine, remedy (Lane iii 940;
Ham 127). 2) معجون "kneaded stuff,
dough; electuary; drugs mixed up
with honey ... generally applied to
such as contains opium, or some
other intoxicating ingredient" (Lane
v 1968; Ham 258). 3) مربا .... fruit
syrup (مراب) thickened by the heat of
the sun or an open fire (KMU 60, 62,
63; ISC v 108, 127; BPK ii 149;
SHA 863 ربّ; Ham 251).
HHP i 1192, ii 1321

(c) RPP 399: "Confections [electuaries,
conserves] are saccharine, soft mas-
ses, in which one or more medicinal
substances are incorporated with the

object of providing an agreeable form
of their administration, and a convenient method for their administration, and a convenient method for
their preservation ... These preparations have been in use for
centuries."
DUS 325
HHP i 1192
دواء Ham 127-135, مربّى Ham 251-253,
معجون Ham 258-292.

Musk   مسك, مسكر מור
155r 16; 155v 2, 12

(o) The Hebrew and Latin translations
רפואת המור הקר and *medicinae
musci* do not correspond to the
Arabic text دواء المسك البارد.

(a) Dozy ii 668 "مسكّر *muskir* pour l'hébreu
שֵׁכָר, boisson enivrante."
See there various sources.

(b) SHA 1872 مسكّر *musakkar* préparation
enivrante.
See *Musk* also in the lists of *Animals
and Animal Products* and *Plants and
Plant Products*.

Oil   دهن שמן
142r 7; 156v 1

(a) Lane iii 926: Oil, sometimes an ingredient of, or serves as ointment.
ZTa 78: "The fatness or oily essence...
extracted from certain substances by
pharmaceutical processes ... being
the vital constituent for medicinal
use."
DUS I 39 *Oleum Amygdalae Amarae*.
"Bitter Almond Oil is the volatile oil
obtained from the dried ripe kernels
of *Prunus Amygdalus Batsch*, or
from other kernels obtaining amyg-
dalin."
HHP i 411, 417; Ergänz.bd. I 206,
207, II i 490

(b) ZTa 81, 90 (tr. 98, 114) دهن زيت the
olive oil. 82, 90, 91 (tr. 101, 115)
دهن اللوز the duhn of almond.
SHA 828

Oxymel سكنجبين سكنجبين
137r 10; 152v 1; 151v 17; 155v 5

(a) Dozy i 669
HHP ii 153
Ham 165

(b) ISC v 108-113
Schm 395

(c) DUS I 814: "The British pharmacopoeia recognizes oxymel as a mixture
of 15 percent each of acetic acid and
distilled water in purified honey."
HHP ii 153: Mentions different
formulas for oxymel.
Ham 165-166

Preserves مربّا ,... ,ربّ مرקחת
See also Rob דבש גם ראה
See Medicament.
See also Rob.

Rob ربّ דבש
146r 4, 10; 147r 1; 147v 3, 13

(a) ZTa 136: "A medicated jelly of fruit."
"The inspissated juice of ripe fruit,
with or without honey or sugar, is
boiled to the consistency of a con-
serve."
ISC v 108: Rob is, by its nature, a thick
juice, and even the syrup is prepared
from decoctions or juices, their
thickness is caused by the sweet stuff.
Ham 136: "The extract of a fruit "rub"
is obtained by regulated concentra-
tion of a fruit or vegetable juice either
with or without the addition of
sugar".
THP II i 43

(b) KMU 60, 62
ISC v 108-9, 127-8
ISC v 109, 127
KMU 60, 62
SHA 863

(c) ZTa 136: Used also (by al-Zahrāwī) as
vehicles instead of honey for blend-
ing medicines.
Ham 136-138

See also the list of *Animals and Animal
Products:* Honey (p. 226).

Sweetmeats حلواء מתיקה
153r 14

(a) Lane ii 634: Sweetmeat, also sweet
fruits
Ham 115-118
KS 110: No sweet fruits in general. 79
translates: sweet dates.

(c) Ham *ibid.*

Syrup شراب משקה
See also Drink, Wine. יין גם ראה

Vinegar خلّ חומץ
150v 13; 152r 1; 156v 6

(a) Lane ii 779: Cites many particulars of
its sources, qualities, applications,
even medical ones.
HHP i 99, 101; ii 1299; Ergänz.bd. I
86; II i 365

(b) SHA 762

(c) RPP 330: "Vinegars form an old class
of preparations, having been in use
since the days of Hippocrates. Medicated vinegars are solutions of the
active principles of drugs in dilute
acetic acid, the latter being chosen as
a menstruum because it is not only
a good solvent, but also possesses
antiseptic properties."

Wine شراب ,خمر יין
See also Drink, Syrup משקה גם ראה
**133r 10; 134r 1, 5; 134v 16; 135r 4;
150r 6; 151r 11, 16; 151v 1, 4, 5, 7;
152r 1, 10; 152v 4; 153v 17; 154r 3,
11, 16; 154v 4, 8; 155r 2, 6; 155v 10,
14; 156v 6**

(o) The Arabic sources distinguish between خمر wine, the matter and شراب
the medical drink.

(a) شربت Ham 169
خمر HHP ii 910, 914 *Vinum;* Ergänz.-
bd. I 1149, II i 1961

(b) KMU 60, 62: شراب one of composed
liquid remedies.

247

SHA 769

(c)   RPS 1342: "Wine, when generally referred to in pharmacy, means grape wine as is practically the only kind of wine used for pharmaceutical purposes.

Wine as such . . . has some therapeutic and physiological value in its action on digestive, respiratory, cardiovascular, and other reactions in the human body."
Ham 169-189, 314-315

BIBLIOGRAPHY

Adams, Francis. *See* Hippocrates; Paulus Aegineta.

Aristotle. *Sleep and Wakefulness.* (De somno et vigilia). Being part of the *Parva naturalia,* 453^b 11–458^a 3. *In*: William David Ross, ed. *The Works of Aristotle.* vol. 3. Oxford, 1931, reprinted 1955.

—. *Problems* [Problemata]. 859^a 1–967^b 27. *In:* William David Ross, ed. *The Works of Aristotle.* vol. 7. Oxford, 1927, reprinted 1953.

Arora, R.B. "Cardiovascular Pharmotherapeutics of Six Medicinal Plants Indigenous to Pakistan and India." *Hamdard,* 12 (1969): 421f.

Avicenna (Ibn Sīnā) *The Canon of Medicine.* Latin translation by Gerard of Cremona, Venice, 1593 (1st ed., Milan, 1476). Hebrew translation by Nathan ha-Meati and Joseph ben Joshua II (Ibn Vives) al-Lorqi, Naples, 1491–1492. English translation of the first book by Oskar Cameron Gruner, London, 1930. German translation of the fifth book by Joseph von Sontheimer, Freiburg, 1845.

—. *De viribus cordis,* sive *De medicinis cordialibus.* Appended to the *Canon,* Padua, 1479, and to some of the later editions.

—. On *De viribus cordis, see* Siddiqi, H.H. and Aziz, M.A.

Ayalon, David and Shin'ar, Pessah. *Milon 'Aravi-'Ivri la-lashon ha'aravit heḥadasha.* 4th ed. Jerusalem, 1965. [A modern Arabic-Hebrew dictionary].

Baneth, David Hartwig. *Mose ben Maimon epistulae.* Fasciculus I. Jerusalem, 1946. [Hebrew and Arabic].

Bar-Sela, Ariel; Hoff, Hebbel E.; and Faris, Elias, eds. "Moses Maimonides' Two Treatises on the Regimen of Health." Translated from the Arabic, . . . etc. *Transactions of the American Philosophical Society.* New Series, 54 (1964): Part 4.

Beit-Arié, Malachi. "An Unknown Translation of Maimonides' Medical Works." *Kirjath Sepher* 38 (1962–1963): 567–574. [In Hebrew].

—. "Codicologic Features as Palaeographic Criteria in Medieval Hebrew MSS." *Kirjath Sepher* 45 (1969–1970): 435–466. [In Hebrew].

Berendes, Julius. *Die Pharmazie bei den alten Kulturvölkern.* 2 vols. Halle, 1891; reprinted Hildesheim, 1965.

—. "Die Hausmittel des Pedanios Dioskurides." *Janus* 12 (1907): 10–33, 79–102, 140–163, 203–224, 268–292, 340–350, 401–412.

Bibliothecae Bodleianae codicum manuscriptorum orientalium Catalogus, I. Oxford, 1787.

Björkman, Walther. *Beiträge zur Geschichte der Staatskanzlei im islamischen Aegypten.* Hamburg, 1928.

Bodenheimer, Fritz Simon. *Ergebnisse der Sinai-Expedition 1927*. Leipzig, 1929.

Brockelmann, Carl. *Geschichte der Arabischen Litteratur*. 2 vols. and *Supplement*, Weimar, 1898–1902; 3 vols., Leiden, 1937–1942.

Caelius Aurelianus. *On Acute and on Chronic Diseases*. Edited and translated by Israel Edward Drabkin. Chicago, 1950.

Castellus, Bartholomaeus. *Lexicon medicum graeco-latinum*. Geneva, 1746. (First edition: *Totius artis medicae, methodo divisiva compendium, et synopsis*. Messina, 1597).

Celsus. *De medicina*. Translated by Walter George Spencer. 3 vols. London and Cambridge, Mass., 1935–1938. (Loeb Classical Library).

Clément-Mullet, M. "Essai sur la minéralogie arabe." *Journal asiatique* 11 (1868): 5–81, 109–253, 502–522.

Ad-Damîrî's Ḥayât al-Ḥayawân. (A zoological lexicon). Translated by A.S.G. Jayakar. vol. i and vol. ii Pt. 1. London and Bombay, 1906–1908.

Dana, Edward Salisbury and Ford, William E., eds. *A Textbook of Mineralogy*. 4th ed. New York, 1957.

Daremberg, Charles. *See* Galen; Rufus.

De Biberstein Kazimirski, Albin. *Dictionnaire arabe-français*. 2 vols. Paris, 1860.

Dierbach, Johann Heinrich. *Die Arzneimittel des Hippocrates*. Heidelberg, 1824; reprinted Hildesheim, 1969.

Dietrich, Albert. *Medicinalia Arabica*. Göttingen, 1966.

Dioscorides. *De materia medica*. Editions used: (a) Greek with Latin translation by Kurt Sprengel, Leipzig, 1829–1830; (b) Greek text edited by Max Wellmann, 3 vols., Berlin, 1907–1914; (c) German translation by Julius Berendes, Stuttgart, 1902; reprinted Wiesbaden, 1970. (d) English translation by John Goodyer (1655), edited by Robert William Theodore Gunther, Oxford, 1934 and New York, 1959; (e) Spanish translation by César Emil Dubler, 6 vols., Barcelona, 1953–1959; (f) Latin translation by Joannes Ruellius, Lyons, 1552.

—. *See* Berendes, Julius. "Die Hausmittel . . .". 1907.

The Dispensatory of the U.S.A. Edited by Arthur Osol, George Elbert Farrer. 24th ed. Philadelphia, 1950.

Dor, Menahem. *Zoological lexicon. Vertebrata*. Tel-Aviv, 1965. [In Hebrew].

Dozy, Reinhart. *Supplément aux dictionnaires arabes*. Leyden, Paris, 1881; 2nd ed., 2 vols., 1927.

Dragendorff, Georg. *Die Heilpflanzen der verschiedenen Völker and Zeiten*. Stuttgart, 1898; reprinted München, 1967.

Du Cange, Charles. *Glossarium mediae et infimae latinitatis*. 10 vols. in 5. Niort, 1883–1887; reprinted Graz, 1954.

Ducros, M.A.H. *Essai sur le droguier populaire arabe de l'inspectorat des pharmacies du Caire*. Cairo, 1930. (Mémoires présentés à l'Institut d'Égypte . . . Tome 15).

Economo, Constantin von. "Schlaftheorie." *In:* L. Asher und K. Spiro, eds. *Ergebnisse der Physiologie* 28 (1929): 312–339.

Eig, Alexander; Zohary, Michael; and Feinbrun, Noemi. *Analytical flora of Palestine.* 2nd ed. Jerusalem, 1965. [In Hebrew].

Encyclopaedia of Islam. Houtsma, Martijn Theodoor., et al., eds. 4 vols. and suppl. Leyden-London, 1913–1938; new edition edited by Hamilton Alexander Rosskeen Gibb et al., Leyden-London, 1960–.

[*Ethics of the Fathers*]. *Sayings of the Jewish Fathers. See*: Taylor, Charles.

Faber, Johann Ernst. De manna ebraeorum opuscula. *In:* I.I. Reiske et J.E. Faber. *Opuscula medica ex monimentis arabum et ebraeorum.* Halle, 1776. *See* Reiske, I.I.

Falaqera, Shem-Tob. *Ha-mebakkesh.* The Hague, 1778. [In Hebrew].

Farmer, Henry George. "Maimonides on Listening to Music". *Journal of the Royal Asiatic Society* 1933, 867–884. Republished with additions in *Mediaeval Jewish tracts on Music.* Vol. I, Bearsden, 1941.

Feliks, Yehuda. *Plant World of the Bible.* 2nd ed. Ramat Gan, 1968. [In Hebrew].

Ferrarius de Gradibus, Johannes Matthaeus. *See* Maimonides, *Regimen.*

Friedenwald, Harry. *Jewish Luminaries in Medical History and a Catalogue.* Baltimore, 1946.

Gärtner, Hans. *See* Rufus of Ephesus.

Galen.* *Opera omnia.* Greek text with Latin translation, edited by Carolus Gottlob Kühn. 20 vols. (in 22). Leipzig, 1821–1833.

—. *Oeuvres anatomiques, physiologiques et médicales de Galien.* Translated by Charles Daremberg. 2 vols. Paris, 1854–1856.

—. *Werke des Galenos.* Trans. Erich Beintker and Wilhelm Kahlenberg. iii and iv. Stuttgart, 1948 and 1952.

—. *De sanitate tuenda.* Translated by Robert Montraville Green. Springfield, Ill., 1951.

—. *Galen on the Usefulness of the Parts of the Body.* Translated by Margaret T. May. 2 vols. Ithaca, N.Y., 1968.

—. *On the natural faculties.* Translated by Arthur J. Brock. London and Cambridge, Mass., 1928. (Loeb Classical Library).

—. *De consuetudinibus.* 1) Greek editions by Friedrich Reinhold Dietz, Leipzig, 1832, and by Iwan Mueller, in *Scripta Minora*, vol. II, 9–31, Leipzig, 1891; 2) Latin translation by Iwan Mueller, Erlangen, 1879; 3) French translation by Charles Daremberg, in *Oeuvres . . . de Galien.* I, 92–110, Paris, 1854; 4) German translation from Hunayn's version by Franz Pfaff, in *Corpus Medicorum Graecorum*, Supplementum.3, Leipzig and Berlin, 1941. *See also:* Konrad Schubring in his "*Bemerkungen zu der Galenausgabe . . . etc.*", inserted in Kühn's *Galeni Opera Omnia*, vol. XX, pp. LV–LVI, reprinted, Hildesheim, 1965.

—. *Die säfteverdünnende Diät. In: Werke des Galenos.* Translated by Erich Beintker and Wilhelm Kahlenberg. iii and iv, Stuttgart, 1948 and 1952.

---

* This reference covers the titles mentioned in this volume. Only special editions and translations or items not included in Kühn's edition are listed separately.

Gaon, Moshe David. [*Oriental Jews in Eretz Israel*]. 2 vols. Jerusalem, 1938. [In Hebrew].

Gesenius, Wilhelm, et al. *Hebräisches und aramäisches Handwörterbuch über das Alte Testament*. Edited by Frantz Buhl. 17th ed. Leipzig, 1921.

Goltz, Dietlinde. *Studien zur Geschichte der Mineralnamen in Pharmazie, Chemie und Medizin von den Anfängen bis Paracelsus*. Wiesbaden, 1972. (*Sudhoffs Archiv*. Beihefte. Heft 14).

Goss, Charles Mayo. "On Anatomy of Veins and Arteries by Galen of Pergamos." *Anatomical Record* 141 (1961): 355–366.

Grzimek, Bernhard et al. *Grzimeks Tierleben*. Enzyclopädie des Tierreiches. 13 vols. Zürich, 1967–1972.

Gurlt, Ernst Julius. *Geschichte der Chirurgie*. 3 vols. Berlin, 1898.

Haebler, Konrad. *Die deutschen Buchdrucker des XV. Jahrhunderts im Auslande*. München, 1924.

Hager's Handbuch der Pharmazeutischen Praxis. 2 vols. and *Ergänzungsband*. 3rd ed. Berlin, 1949; 2. *Ergänzungsband*. 2 vols., 1958.

Halevi, Judah. *Poems*. Translated from Hebrew: (a) into German by Abraham Geiger, *Divan des Abu'l-Hassan Juda ha-Levi*, Breslau, 1851, and by Franz Rosenzweig, *Jehuda Halevi, Zweiundneunzig Hymnen und Gedichte*. 2nd ed., Berlin, 1925; (b) into English by Nina Salaman, *Selected Poems of Jehuda Halevi*, London, 1924; reprinted Philadelphia, 1946.

Hamdard: Pharmacopoeia of Eastern Medicine. Said Hakim Mohammed, ed. *Hamdard. The Organ of the Institute of Health and Tibbi Research*. 12 (1969): nos. 1–4.

Heberden, William. *Antitheriaca: An Essay on Mithridatium and Theriaca*. London, 1745.

Hippocrates. *Works*. Translated by William Henry Samuel Jones. 4 vols. London and Cambridge, Mass., 1923, reprinted 1948. (Loeb Classical Library).

—. *Oeuvres complètes*. Traduction par Émile Littré avec le text grec. 10 vols. Paris, 1839–1861.

—. *The Genuine Works*. Translated by Francis Adams. 2 vols. London, 1849.

Hoppe, H.A. *Drogenkunde*. 7th ed. Hamburg, 1958.

Howell, Jesse V. and Weller, James Martin, eds. *Glossary of Geology and Related Sciences*. 2nd ed. American Geology Institute, Washington, 1962.

Hunnius, Curt. *Pharmazeutisches Wörterbuch*. 4th ed. Berlin, 1966.

Hyrtl, Joseph. *Das Arabische und Hebräische in der Anatomie*. Wien, 1879.

Iamblichos' Life of Pythagoras. Translated by Thomas Taylor. London, 1818.

Ibn al-Bayṭār. *Kitāb al-jāmi'* . . . etc. Translated by Joseph von Sontheimer. *Grosse Zusammenstellung über die Kräfte der bekannten einfachen Heil- und Nahrungsmittel*. 2 vols. Stuttgart, 1840–1842.

Ibn Ezra, Abraham. *Works*. Edited by David Kahana. 2 vols. Warsaw, 1894. [In Hebrew].

Ibn Sīnā. *See* Avicenna.

Irigoin, J. "Les premiers manuscrits grecs écrits sur papier et le problème du bombycin." *Scriptorium* 4 (1950): 194–204.

—. "Les débuts de l'emploi du papier à Byzance." *Byz. Zeitschrift* 46 (1953): 320–324.

Issa Bey, Ahmed. *Dictionnaire des noms des plantes on latin, français, anglais et arabe.* Le Caire, 1930.

Kaiser, Alfred. *Der heutige Stand der Mannafrage.* Arbon, 1924.

Al-Kindī, Abū Yūsuf Yaʿkūb b. Isḥāk. *The medical formulary or Aqrābādhīn of Al-Kindī.* Translated by Martin Levey. Madison, 1966.

Klein-Franke, Felix. "Der hippokratische und maimonidische Arzt." *Freiburger Zeitschr. für Philosophie und Theologie* 17 (1970): 442–449.

Kleitman, Nathaniel. *Sleep and Wakefulness.* 2nd ed. Chicago, 1963. [1434 references].

Klibansky, Raymond; Panofsky, Erwin; and Saxl, Fritz. *Saturn and Melancholy.* London, 1964.

Knaʿani, Yaʿakov. *Oẓar hallašon haʿivrit litekufoteyha hăššonot.* vol. 1–. Jerusalem-Tel-Aviv, 1940–. [Dictionary of the Hebrew language. In Hebrew].

Kraus, Paul. *Jābīr ibn Ḥayyān, II, "La science des propriétiés."* Le Caire, 1942. (Mémoires de l'Institut d'Égypte, 45.)

Kroner, Hermann. *Ein Beitrag zur Geschichte der Medizin des XII. Jahrhunderts.* Oberdorf-Bopfingen, 1906.

—. "Die Haemorrhoiden in der Medizin des XII. and XIII. Jahrhunderts." *Janus* 16 (1914): 441–456, 645–718.

—. "Fī tadbīr aṣ-ṣiḥḥat, Gesundheitsanleitung des Maimonides für den Sultan al-Malīk al-Afḍal." [First edition of the Arabic text, German translation, notes]. *Janus* 21 (1923–1925): 101–116, 286–300; 28: 61–74, 143–152, 199–217, 408–419, 455–472; 29: 235–258.

—. *Der Mediciner Maimonides im Kampfe mit dem Theologen.* Oberdorf-Bopfingen, 1924.

—. "Der medizinische Schwanengesang des Maimonides." [De causis accidentium]. [First edition of the Arabic text, German translation, notes.] *Janus* 32 (1928): 12–116.

On Kroner. See Marcus, Shlomo.

Kümmel, Werner. "Melancholie und die Macht der Musik." *Medizinhistorisches Journal* 4 (1969): 189–209.

Laín Entralgo, Pedro. *La historia clinica.* Madrid, 1950.

Lane, Edward William. *An Arabic-English Lexicon.* Book I, 8 parts. London, 1863–1893.

Leibowitz, Joshua O. "A Probable Case of Peptic Ulcer as Described by Amatus Lusitanus (1556)." *Bull. Hist. Med.* 27 (1953): 212–216.

—. "Book of Medical Experiences Ascribed to Abraham ibn Ezra (1089–1164)." *Harofe Haivri* 26 (1953[b]): 151–159. [In Hebrew with English summary].

—. "Maimonides on Medical Practice." *Bull. Hist. Med.* 31 (1957): 309–317.

—. *The History of Coronary Heart Disease.* London and Berkeley, 1970.

Leveen, Jacob. "Pharmaceutical Fragment of the Tenth Century in Hebrew by Shabbatai Donnolo." *Proc. Roy. Soc. Med., Sect. Hist. Med.* 21 (1927–1928): 67–70.

Levy, Reuben. "The 'Tractatus de Causis et Indicis Morborum' attributed to Maimonides." *In*: Charles Singer, ed. *Studies in the History and Method of Science* 1 (1917): 225–234.

Lexikon-Institut Bertelsmann. *Ich sag dir alles.* Gütersloh, 1966.

Löw, Immanuel. *Aramaeische Pflanzennamen.* Leipzig, 1881.

—. *Die Flora der Juden.* 4 vols. Wien and Leipzig, 1924–1934; reprinted Hildesheim, 1967.

Maimonides. *Aphorisms* [Fuṣūl Mūsā fī aṭ-ṭibb]. Latin editions: Bologna 1489; Venice 1497; Venice 1508; Basel 1579. Hebrew translations: Lemberg 1834; Wilna 1888; Jerusalem 1959 (edited by Süssmann Muntner). English translation: by Fred Rosner and Süssmann Muntner; vol. I (sections 1–14), vol. II (sections 15–25). New York, 1970 ,1971.

—. *Glossary of Materia Medica* [Kitāb sharḥ asmā' al-'uqqār]. *See* Meyerhof, 1940; Muntner, 1969.

—. *The Book on Asthma* [Maḳāla fī ar-rabū]. *See* Muntner, 1940.

—. *Commentary on the Aphorisms of Hippocrates* [Sharḥ fuṣūl Abūḳrāṭ]. *See* Muntner, 1961.

—. *The Guide for the Perplexed* [Dalālat al-ḥā'irīn]. English translations by Michael Friedländer, London 1881–1885; by Shlomo Pines, *The Guide of the Perplexed.* Chicago, 1963.

—. *Mishneh Torah* [Religious Code]. Hebrew and English (Part I only), edited ... and translated by Moses Hyamson. New York, 1937. Some of the other fourteen parts translated into English in the Yale Judaica Series, New Haven 1949–. (General title: *The Code of Maimonides.*)

—. On Poisons [Kitāb as-sumūm wa-al-mutaḥarriz min al-adwiya al-ḳattāla]. For Hebrew medieval translation, see Muntner, 1942; French translation by Israël-Michel Rabbinowicz, Paris, 1865, reprinted 1935.

—. Maimonides' Treatise on Resurrection. [Maḳāla fī teḥiyyat hametīm]. Ed. Joshua Finkel, New York, American Academy for Jewish Research, 1939.

—. *Regimen sanitatis* [Kitāb tadbīr aṣ-ṣiḥḥa]. In Arabic with German translation, *see* Kroner, 1923–1925. Latin editions:

a) Tractatus Rabi Moysi, Florence c. 1477; facsimile of this edition, with preface by Aron Freimann, Heidelberg, 1931;

b) *in*: Ferrarius de Gradibus, *Tabula consiliorum*, Pavia, 1501;

c) *in*: idem, *Consiliorum ... utile repertorium*, Venice, 1514;

d) *Tractatus ... de regimine sanitatis*, ... Augsburg, 1518;

e) *in*: Ferrarius de Gradibus, *Consilia ...* Lyons, 1535;

Hebrew translations: in *Kerem Ḥemed*, Prague 3 (1838): 9–31, Jerusalem, 1885; Jerusalem, 1957 (ed. by Muntner). In English: Philadelphia, 1964 (ed. by Bar-Sela, Hoff and Faris), *in*: *Trans. Amer. Phil. Soc.*, 1964, New Series, 54, Part 4. In German: Leiden, 1923–1925 (*See* Kroner); Basel, 1966; reprinted 1969 (*See* Muntner).

—. *De causis accidentium* [Maqālah fī bayān ba'ḍ al-a'rāḍ wa-al-jawāb 'anhā]. *See* Kroner, *Der medizinische Schwanengesang* etc., 1928; Bar-Sela et al., *Moses Maimonides, Two Treatises* etc., 1964; Muntner, *Medical Responses* etc., 1966.

—. Benamara, Joseph, '*De causis accidentium*'. Medical thesis, Strasbourg, 1973.

—. Epistulae. *See* Baneth, 1946.

Marcus, Shlomo. "Hermann Kroner". [A bio-bibliography]. *Koroth* 5 (1971): 681–688 [in Hebrew], xcvi–xcix [in English].

May, Margaret T. "On Translating Galen". *J. Hist. Med.* 25 (1970): 168–176.

—. *See: Galen on the Usefulness of the Parts of the Body*, 1968.

Merck's Warenlexicon für Handel, Industrie und Gewerbe. Edited by Adolf Beythien, M. Arnold and Ernst Dressler. 7th ed. Leipzig, 1920.

Meyerhof, Max. "Über das Leidener arabische Fragment von Galen's Schrift 'Über die medizinischen Namen'." *Sitz. Preuss. Akad. Wiss.*, (Phil. Hist. Kl.) 23 (1928): 296–319.

—. "L'oeuvre médicale de Maïmonide." *Archeion* 9 (1929): 136–155.

—. *Šarḥ asmā' al-'uqqār (L'explication des noms de drogues). Un glossaire de matière médicale composé par Maïmonide.* Texte, trad. et comm. Le Caire, 1940.

Mielck, R. *Terminologie und Technologie der Müller und Bäcker im islamischen Mittelalter.* (Inaugural-Dissertation). Hamburg, 1914.

Morgagni, Giovanni Battista. *De sedibus et causis morborum per anatomen indagatis.* Padua, 1761.

Muntner, Süssmann. *Moshe ben Maimon. Medical Works*:

— —. *The Book on Asthma.* Jerusalem. 1940 (Sefer haqqazzeret o sefer hammis'adim). [Maḳāla fī ar-rabū].

—. —. *Poisons and Their Antidotes or "The Treatise to the Honoured One".* Jerusalem. 1942. (Samme hammawet weharefu'ot kenegdam o "hamma'amar hanikhbad"). [Kitāb as-sumūm wa-al-mutaḥarriz min al-adwiya al-ḳattāla].

—. —. *Regimen sanitatis.* Jerusalem. 1957. (Hanhagat habberi'ut). [Kitāb tadbīr aṣ-ṣiḥḥa].

—. —. *(Medical) Aphorisms of Moses.* Jerusalem, 1959. (Pirke Moshe (birefu'a)). [Fuṣūl Mūsā fī aṭ-ṭibb].

—. —. *Commentary on Hippocrates' Aphorisms.* Jerusalem, 1961. (Perush lepirke Abuqraṭ). [Sharḥ fuṣūl Abūḳrāṭ].

—. —. *On Hemorrhoids.* Jerusalem, 1965. (Birefu'at hattehorim). [Risāla fī al-bawāsīr].

—. —. *Lexicography of Drugs.* (Be'ur shemot harefu'ot). [Kitāb sharḥ asmā' al-'uḳḳār]. Modern Hebrew translation, based on Meyerhof's edition. Bound with

—. —. *Medical Responses.* (Teshuwot refu'iyot). [Maḳāla fī bayān ba'ḍ al-a'rāḍ]. Being *De causis accidentium* (Ma'amar hahakhra'a). Jerusalem, 1969.

—. *Regimen sanitatis . . . mit Anhang der Medizinischen Responsen und Ethik des Maimonides.* Deutsche Übersetzung. Basel. 1966; reprinted 1969.

Muwaffak [Muwaffaq], Abū Manṣūr. "Die pharmakologischen Grundsätze." Translated by Abdul Chalig Achundow. *In: Kobert's Historische Studien aus dem Pharmakologischen Institute der Universität Dorpat* 3 (1893): 113–414, 450–481; reprinted Leipzig, 1968.

Neubauer, Adolf. *Facsimiles of Hebrew Manuscripts in the Bodleian Library.* Oxford, 1886.

—. *Catalogue of the Hebrew Manuscripts in the Bodleian Library.* Oxford, 1886–1906.

Neave, S.A. *Nomenclator zoologicus.* 4 vols. London. 1939–1940. vols. 5, 6 1950–1966.

Paulus Aegineta. *The Seven Books.* Translation and commentary by Francis Adams. 3 vols. London, 1844–1847.

Paulys Real — Encyclopädie der classischen Altertumswissenschaft . . . Herausgegeben von Georg Wissowa. vol. 1 —. Stuttgart, 1894–.

Pavlov, Ivan Petrovich. *Lectures on the Principal Digestive Glands.* In Russian: Petersburg, 1897; English translation by William Henry Thompson titled *The Work of the Digestive Glands*, London, 1902.

Peters, Hans. *Lehrbuch der Mineralogie und Geologie.* 2nd ed. Kiel und Leipzig, 1905.

"Picatrix" Das Ziel des Weisen von Pseudo-Maǧrīṭī. Arabic text edited by Hellmut Ritter. Leipzig, 1933.

—. German translation by Hellmut Ritter and Martin Plessner, London, 1962.

Piéron, Henri. *Le problème physiologique du sommeil.* Paris, 1913.

Pliny. *Natural History.* Translated by Harris Rackham and others. 10 vols. London and Cambridge, Mass., 1938–1963. (Loeb Classical Library).

Portaleone, Abraham. *De auro dialogi tres . . . de specifica ejus forma.* Venice, 1584.

Post, George E. *Flora of Syria, Palestine and Sinai.* 2 vols. 2nd ed. Beirut, 1932–1933.

The School of Salernum. Regimen sanitatis Salerni. English version by Sir John Harington. Salerno, [no date].

Reiske, Ioannes Iacobus et Faber, Ioannes Ernestus. *Opuscula medica ex monimentis arabum et ebraeorum.* Halle, 1776.

Relandus, Hadrianus. *Palaestina ex monumentibus ulteribus illustrata.* Utrecht, 1714.

Remington's Pharmaceutical Sciences. Edited by A. Osol, a.o. 14th ed. Easton, 1970.

Remington's Practice of Pharmacy. Edited by Eric Wontworth Martin and Ernest Fullerton Cook. 11th ed. Easton, 1956.

Richter, Paul. "Beiträge zur Geschichte des Aussatzes." *Sudhoffs Archiv* 4 (1910): 323–352.

Rosner, Fred. *See* Maimonides. *Aphorisms.*

Rufinus. *The Herbal of Rufinus.* Edited by Lynn Thorndike and Francis S. Benjamin. Chicago, 1946.

Rufus of Ephesus. Greek text with French translation by Charles Daremberg and Ch. Émile Ruelle. Paris, 1879.

—. *Die Fragen des Arztes an den Kranken:* herausgegeben, übersetzt und erläutert von Hans Gärtner. Berlin, 1962. (Corpus medicorum graecorum, supplementum IV).

Ruska, Julius, ed. and transl. *Das Steinbuch aus der Kosmographie des Zakarijâ ibn Muḥammad ibn Maḥmûd al-Kazwînî.* Beilage zum Jahresbericht 1895-6 der prov. Oberrealschule. Heidelberg, 1896.

—. ed. and transl. *Das Steinbuch des Aristoteles.* Heidelberg, 1912.

Schedel, H. "Die Gewürzkonfekte und Weine als Schutz- und Geschmacksmittel bei der Mahlzeit auf der Reise und in Wirtshäusern." *Archiv für Gesch. der Medizin* 13 (1921): 171–172.

Schery, Robert Walter. *Plants for man.* New-York, 1952. (Prentice-Hall Plant Science Series).

Schmucker, Werner. *Die pflanzliche und mineralische materia medica im Firdaus al-Hikma des Tabarī.* Bonn, 1969. (Bonner Orientalistische Studien, Neue Serie, 18).

Schweinfurth, Georg. *Arabische Pflanzennamen aus Aegypten, Algerien und Jemen.* Berlin, 1912.

Seidel, Ernst. "Die Medizin im Kitâb Mafâtîḥ al 'Ulûm." *Sitzungsber. phys. med. Sozietät, Erlangen* 47 (1915): 1–79.

Shlamovitz, Naomi, *The pharmacological properties of extracts from the plants Anchusa strigosa and Echium amoenum (Fam. Boraginaceae).* M. Sc. thesis, Tel Aviv University, 1973.

Siddiqi, H.H. and Aziz, M.A. "A Note on Avicenna's Tract on Cardiac Drugs." *Planta Medica. Zeitschr. für Arzneipflanzenforsch.* 11 (1963). Heft 4.

Siggel, Alfred. *Arabisch-Deutsches Wörterbuch der Stoffe aus den drei Naturreichen.* Berlin, 1950.

Singer, Charles, ed. *Studies in the History and Method of Science.* Oxford, Vols. I and II. 1917-1921; reprinted 1955.

Spirt, Beverly A. "A Preliminary Study of the Hebrew Text of a Medical Treatise by Maimonides." [Typewritten]. Bachelor's thesis. Harvard University, 1967.

Steingass, Francis Joseph. *A Comprehensive Persian-English Dictionary.* London, 1892.

Steinmetz, E.F. *Codex vegetabilis.* Amsterdam, 1957.

Steinschneider, Moritz. "Gifte und ihre Heilung". *Virchow's Archiv* 57 (1873): 62–120.

—. *Die hebräischen Handschriften der K. Hof- und Staatsbibliothek in München.* München, 1875.

—. *Die hebräischen Übersetzungen des Mittelalters und die Juden als Dolmetscher.* Berlin, 1893; reprinted Graz, 1956.

—. "Die Vorrede des Maimonides zu einem Commentar über die Aphorismen des Hippo-crates." *Zeitschr. Deutsch. Morgenl. Ges.* 48 (1894): 218–234.

—. "Heilmittelnamen der Araber." *Wiener Zeitschr. für Kunde des Morgenlandes* 1897–1899, 11: 259–278, 313–330; 12: 1–20; 13: 75–94.

—. *Die arabische Literatur der Juden.* Frankfurt a/M., 1902.

Sudhoff, Karl. *Kurzes Handbuch der Geschichte der Medizin.* 3rd and 4th eds. Berlin, 1922.

Taylor, Charles, translated and edited. *Sayings of the Jewish Fathers* [Pirke avot, Ethics of the Jewish Fathers]. Cambridge, 1877, 1897. Appendix, 1899.

Teicher, Avishai. *History of Peptic Ulcer.* [Typewritten]. M.D. thesis, Jerusalem, 1970. [Hebrew with English summary].

Tschirch, Alexander. *Handbuch der Pharmakognosie.* 2nd ed. Leipzig, 1932.

Tuḥfat al-aḥbāb. *Glossaire de la matière médicale marocaine.* Edited by Henry Paul Joseph Renaud, Georges Seraphin Colin. Paris, 1934. (Publications de l'Institut des Hautes-Études Marocaines. Tome xxiv.)

UNESCO. *Medicinal Plants of the Arid Zone.* Paris, 1960. (Arid Zone Research. xiii).

Vajda, Georges. *Index général des manuscrits arabes musulmans de la Bibliothèque Nationale.* Paris, 1953.

Vesalius, Andreas. *De humani corporis fabrica.* 2nd ed. Basel, 1555.

Vullers, Johann August. *Lexicon persico-latinum etymologicum.* Bonn, 1855–1867.

Wahrmund, Adolf. *Handwörterbuch der arabischen und deutschen Sprache.* 2 vols. Giessen, 1877.

Watson, Gilbert. *Theriac and Mithridatium: A Study in Therapeutics.* London, 1966.

Wehr, Hans. *Arabisches Wörterbuch.* Wiesbaden, 1958.

Wellmann, Max. "Die φυσικα des Bolos Democritos, *etc.*" *Abh. Preuss. Akad. Wiss.,* Phil. Hist. Kl., No. 7, 1928.

Zaitschek, David Victor. "*Semen Psyllii* . , . from the Judean Desert Caves." [In press].

Zohary Michael. *Flora palaestina.* Jerusalem. Part. i 1966; part. ii 1972.

Zotenberg, Hermann. *Catalogue des manuscrits hébreux et samaritains de la Bibliothèque Nationale.* Paris, 1866. (Manuscrits orientaux, série 1).

INDEX

Abrabanel, Isaac, 101
'Accidens', meaning of, 10
Adam of Fulda, 107
Adams, Francis, 12, 17, 87
al-Afḍal, *Sultan*, 9, 15, 20, 25;
    detailed instructions of daily routine and
    preparation of food and drink for, 111–149;
    regimen to be followed by, 30, 95
al-Fārābī, 160, 161
Alcohol, medical use of, 57, 135, 143.
    See also: Wine, medical use of
'Alī b. al-'Abbās, 115, 117
Alpagus, Andreas, 99
Amatus Lusitanus, 71
Amber, medical use of, 97
American Philosophical Society, 8
Ancient medicine, 51, 53, 67
Animal fats, 119, 123
Appetite, 79, 125
Aristotle (Pseudo-): *De somno et vigilia*, 25;
    Problemata, 107
Arteriosclerosis, 149
Arthritis, 26
Astringent, 83, 119, 131
Atra bilis, 49, 115. *See also:* Bile, black
Aurum Potabile. *See:* Gold, medical use of
Avicenna (Ibn Sīnā), 19, 21, 22, 27, 30, 31, 95,
    103; *Canon*, 16, 33, 47, 99, 105, 106, 139, 160,
    161; *De viribus cordis*, 16, 25, 26, 97, 99, 105,
    111

Balm gentle, medical use of, 21, 111
Barberry, medical use of, 21, 69
Barley, medical use of, 32, 147–150
Barley water, medical use of, 21, 71, 73
Bar-Sela, Ariel, 8, 13, 113, 155, 158, 198
Bathing, 21, 24, 26, 65, 93, 139–141, 147
Beit-Arié, Malachi, 8
Berendes, Julius: 'Die Hausmittel des Pedanios
    Dioskurides', 69

Bible, 101, 129
Bile: black, 20, 23; inflammation of, 67, 91;
    yellow, 20, 63, 65
Biliary conditions, 63
Bibliothèque Nationale, Paris, 13
Blood: corruption and clarification, 14, 23, 53,
    89; exsudation from vessels, 45; hemorrhage,
    45–51; letting, *see:* Venesection; natural or
    good, 19, 55, 89; supposed origination in the
    liver, 14; 'thickness', 14, 20, 22–23, 83–85;
    turbidity and sediment, 45
Bodenheimer, Fritz Simon, 100
Brain, 32, 59, 93; ascent to, 75, 149
Bread: in diet, 113; made white, 28; white or
    coarse, 113

Caelius Aurelianus, 106
Cardamon of Bawa, 101
Cardiac remedies, 16, 25, 31, 77, 91, 99–103, 137
Cardiac symptoms, 16, 27–28, 31, 93, 99, 107
Cardiology, 26
Castoreum, medical use of, 26, 31, 103, 105, 145
Catarrh, 23, 24, 119. *See also:* Phlegm
Celsus: *De medicina*, 27, 107
Chicken broth, medical use of, 115
Coitus, 24, 31, 93, 141–143, 145
Commentary, running, 41–153; its aim, 17
Consilia, 10, 16, 19
Constipation, 19, 20, 150
Coriander, medical use of, 22, 75, 77
Coronary artery disease, 15–16, 99–98
Coronary disease, 16, 103, 106, 149. *See also.*
    Cardiac symptoms
Crab, medical use of, 109
Crisis, 47

Dāwūd al-ḥakīm, 158
Depression. *See:* Melancholia
Diet, 23, 28–30, 79, 81, 113, 115, 117, 119, 121,
    123, 125, 131; according to season, 31, 89,

121–123; dishes, 29–30, 119–125; in animal feeding, 115. *See also:* Maimonides: *Mishneh Torah*

Dietary rules, 67

Dietrich, Albert, 157

Digestion, 21, 53, 59, 61, 67, 73, 143

Digestive disorders, 16

'Dilation of the spirit'. *See:* Oxtongue, medical use of

Dill, medical use of, 149

Dioscorides, 15, 19, 51, 67, 75

Donnolo, Sabbatai, 127

Drugs, 15, 21, 30, 55, 69, 91, 127, 137, 215; cumulative action, 23; habituation, 20, 24, 91–93; precise weights and measures, 53; sympathetic, 24, 27, 91, 98, 101; toxic, 69, 71, 77, 87

Dyscrasia, 47, 117; cardiac, 77

Economo, Constantin von, 25

Ederi, H., 51

Editions of the treatise, 9–13; present multilingual, 17

Eggplant, in diet, 81

Egypt, use of drugs, 25, 57

Electuary, 91, 97, 123, 135, 145; cardiac, 25, 26; jacinth, 16, 26, 27, 31, 99–98, 143. *See also:* Medicaments

Emerald, medical use of, 24, 91

Emetics, 23, 83

Epithymum, 27

Exercise, 21, 24, 25, 31, 65, 81, 93, 95, 131, 139, 143–147

'Exhilarating drink', 19, 21, 53, 91. *See also:* Oxtongue

Falaqera, Shemtob: *Hamebakesh*, 69

Faris, Elias, 13

Farmer, Henry George, 133

Ferrarius de Gradibus, J.M.: *Tabula consiliorum*, 10; *Tractatus quinque*, 10

Fever, 67, 79, 81, 85, 93, 99

Fleabane, medical use of, 21, 69–71

Florentine manuscript, 7, 10, 25

Food spoiling as cause of "putrid fevers", 22, 79–81

Friedenwald, Harry, 8

Friedenwald Collection, Jerusalem, 11, 198

Friedenwald manuscript, 8, 11, 25

Fruit, in diet, 22, 61, 79–81, 131; citrus, 121; soft: rejection on Galen's authority, 22, 79–81

Galen, 13, 14, 19, 20, 31, 32, 49, 55, 59, 79, 89, 113, 125; *Ad Pisonem de Theriaca*, 26; *Adversus Lycum libellus*, 83; *Commentary on Hippocrates on Fractures*, 124; *De alimentorum facultatibus*, 22, 28, 113, 125; *De atra bile*, 14; *De compositione medicamentorum secundum locos*, 27; *De constitutione artis medicae*, 31; *De consuetudinis*, 15; *De differentiis febrium*, 14; *De locis affectis*, 15; *De methodo medendi*, 20, 141; *De naturalibus facultatibus*, 24, 30, 91; *De probis pravisque alimentorum succis*, 22, 81; *De sanitate tuenda*, 14, 25, 81, 115, 127; *De simplicium medicamentorum temperamentis*, 24, 51, 71, 75; *De temperamentis*, 23; *De usu partium*, 14, 93; *Die säfteverdünnende Diät*, 29; *Hippocratis de acutorum morborum victu commentarius*, 14; *In Hippocratis Epid. VI et Galeni in illum commentarius V*, 23; *On Medical Nomenclature*, 63; *On the Natural Faculties*, 53

Gastritis, 73, 113, 119. *See also:* Hyperacidity

Gold, medical use of, 24, 26, 27, 91, 99, 101

Goldschmidt, Ernst Daniel, 8

Greek medicine, 13

Grossberger, Herbert, 7

Hayyim Bekor ha-Levi (Gilibi) ben Ephraim, 9, 34

Heberden, William: *Antitheriaca*, 27

Hebrew script, 35

Hematology, 20, 89

Hemoconcentration, 14, 22–23, 81–83, 147

Hemodilution, 89

Hemorrhoids, 19, 45–51; conservative therapy, 51; surgery in selected cases, 49

Herbs, in diet, 28; medical use of, 27. For individual plants, *see* respective entries, and Materia medica

Hippocrates, 13, 21, 30, 32, 73, 125, 131, 147, 150; *Aphorisms*, 14, 17, 49, 107, 139; *De diaeta*, 29; *On Ancient Medicine*, 13; *On Hemorrhoids*, 49; *Prognostics*, 43; *Regimen in Acute Diseases*, 28, 32, 125, 139, 149; *Sacred Disease*, 15

Historical medicine, terminology in, 45

Hiwi al Balki, 100

Hoff, Hebbel E., 13
Humoral theory, 20, 22, 27, 59, 143
Humors, 47, 67, 149; black, 28, 32, 113, 149
Hydromel, medical use of, 30, 31, 125–129, 131, 139
Hygiene, 65
Hyoscyamus, 27
Hyperacidity, 21, 32, 137, 150. *See also:* Gastritis
Hyrtl, Joseph, 45

Ibn al-Bayṭār, 19, 21, 32, 51, 71, 75, 83, 109
Ibn al-Tilmīdh, 69
Ibn Ezra, Abraham, 101–100; *Book of (Medical) Experiences,* 24, 109; "Regimen of Health" (poem), 67
Ibn Rushd, 29
Ibn Sīnā. *See:* Avicenna
Ibn Zuhr, Abū Marwān, 30, 33, 55; *De nutrimentis,* 22, 29, 79
Ilan, Ilay, 8
Indian medicine, 24
Inflammation, 47, 63, 83, 91
Intoxication, 71
Italian script, 35

Jacinth, medical use of. *See:* Electuary, jacinth
Jacob, Ernst, 8
Jaundice, 29, 107
Jewish National and University Library, Jerusalem, 9, 34, 160
John of Capua, 11, 198
Joseph ben Judah, 12
Judah ha-Levi: "The Physician" (poem), 151
Julep, medical use of, 28, 109

Kabbala, 34
Kaiser, Alfred, 100
Karaite writing, 35
Klein-Franke, Felix, 8, 152
Kleitman N.: *Sleep and Wakefulness,* 25
Klibansky, R. et al.: *Saturn and Melancholy,* 107
Koran, 41
Kroner, Hermann, 12, 35, 71, 73, 115, 147, 150, 152, 155, 157–162, 198
Kümmel, Werner, 107

Laín Entralgo, Pedro: *La historia clinica,* 16
Lapis lazuli, medical use of, 83
Leibowitz, Joshua O., 14, 20, 71, 98, 106, 151

Leprosy, 115, 117
Levy, Reuben, 159
Lieber, Elinor, 7
Lipothymia, 16, 26. *See also:* Coronary disease
Littmann, Enno, 156
Liver, 14, 20, 23, 65, 89

Maimonides: *Aphorisms,* 12, 13, 25, 28, 32, 47, 49, 57, 67, 105, 113, 119, 131; belief in therapy, 152–153; *Book of Poisons,* 25, 158, 159, 161; *Commentary on the Aphorisms of Hippocrates,* 13–14, 157, 158; *De causis accidentium,* 7. 9, 11–12, 159, 160, 198; *Guide for the Perplexed,* 12; headings of works not given by himself, 11, 12, 13, 41; *Mishneh Torah,* 12, 23, 25, 29, 79, 93, 119, 133, 145, 151; *On Coitus,* 35, 37, 159; *On Hemorrhoids,* 45, 47, 49, 158–160; *On Poisons,* 97; *Regimen of Health,* 7, 9–13, 15, 20–23, 25, 28, 35, 65, 67, 79, 113, 147, 157, 158, 159, 198; share in transmission of Greek medicine, 13; *Treatise of Decision,* 11, 16, 41; *Treatise of Resurrection,* 160; *Treatise on Asthma,* 35, 37, 43, 95, 147, 153, 159
Mainz, Ernest, 13, 159
Mania, 107–106
Manic-depressive syndrome, 16, 27, 107–106
Manna, medical use of, 101–100
Manuscript description: Arabic, 155–163; Hebrew, 34–38; Latin, 198–199. *See also:* Texts, Translations
Marcus, Shlomo, 7; 'Hermann Kroner', 12
Marmor, Beverly (née Spirt): "Preliminary study of the Hebrew text of a medical treatise by Maimonides", 7
Materia medica, 215–248: Animals and animal products, 225–229; Hebrew terms, list of, 219–222; Medicaments and foods, 245–248; Mineral substances, 223–225; Plants and plant products, 229–244
Mauthner, L., 25
May, Margaret T.: 'On Translating Galen', 113
Meat, in diet, 28, 81, 89, 113, 115, 117, 119, 123, 125
Mechoulam, Raphael, 51
Medical questioning, art of, 43
Medicaments, 20, 21, 23, 55, 69, 75, 99, 129, 143, 145; cardiac, 24, 30, 91, 125, 137; psychotropic, 91; *versus* nutriments and their

different action, 24, 26, 30, 55, 91, 129. *See also:* Nutrients; Drugs, habituation

Medicine and religion, 29, 32–33, 59, 150–153

Medieval medicine. *See:* Middle Ages, medicine during

Melancholia, 15, 19, 20, 99–98. *See also:* Manic-depressive syndrome

Metabolism, 15, 20, 53, 61, 127, 139; 'the three digestions', 61; unripened matter, 31, 139–143

Meyerhof M., 31, 51, 63, 91, 101, 150, 152, 155, 216

Middle Ages, medicine during, 13, 16, 19, 23, 29, 53, 67, 117, 137, 215, 216

Migraine, 29

Milk, in diet, 21, 67, 115

Minerals, medical use of, 24

Morgagni, Giovanni Battista: *De sedibus et causis morborum*, 45

Morphine, medical use of, 103

Muḥammad ben Aḥmad b. al-'Āṣ al-Andalusī, 158

Muntner, Suessmann,: editions of the medical works of Maimonids, throughout this volume; *Medical Responses*, 12

Music, therapeutic use of, 30, 107, 133–135

Musk, medical use of, 31, 97–99, 143–145

Muwaffak, Abū Manṣūr, 24, 27

Myrrh, 97

Nathan ha-Me'ati, 13, 22

National and University Library, Jerusalem, 8, 9

National Library of Medicine, Bethesda, 8

Nature, 19, 91; expels superfluities, 47–51; healing power of and its limits, 49, 51; natural course of disease, 47–49

Nausea, 77

Neubauer, Adolf, 36, 160

Nutrients, 22, 24, 30, 55, 67, 129

Nutrition, 89, 121; mealtimes, 129; and throughout chapter 20 (111–129)

Odyssey, 125

Opium, medical use of, 21, 26, 32, 103, 147

Oxtongue, medical use of, 15–16, 19, 21, 24, 28, 30–31, 51–59, 85, 109–110, 135; experimental work on, 19, 51, 53

Oxymel, medical use of, 30, 67, 124, 129; of roses, 139, 145

Palaeography, 17, 34–38

Palpitation, 106

Pathophysiology, 17

Paulus Aegineta, 17, 87, 103

Pearls, medical use of, 101

Peptic ulcer, 71, 73

Persian medicine, 24

Petri, Johannes, 10

Pharmacology, 16, 19, 51, 145, 215–216. *See also:* Drugs

Pharmacy, royal, 25, 97

Phlegm, 23–24, 61, 63, 67, 73, 91

Physicians: against interference when nature may help, 49, 53; agreement and disagreement, 43–45, 67–79; 'and philosophers', 30, 133; best or perfect, 16, 43, 55, 57, 83, 97; colleagues, 16, 41; information by history taking, 43, 45; qualities essential for, 153

Physiology: of assimilation, 61, 139; of exercise, 25, 30, 93–95, 131; gastric, 16, 21, 31, 32, 59, 67–73, 123, 135; of hot regions, 81–83 (*see also:* Hemoconcentration); of separation for superfluities, 53; of sleep, 25, 30

Picatrix, 109

Plessner, Martin, 7, 12

Plethora, 23, 87, 89

Pliny, 51

Pocock, Edward, 155

Polycythemia, 14, 15, 23, 87. *See also:* Venesection.

Poppy, medical use of, 71, 73, 147

Portaleone, Abraham, 91, 101

Poultices, 47, 65

Prywes, Moshe, ed., *Israel Journal of Medical Sciences*, 8

Psychiatry, 17

Psychology, 30, 133

Psychopharmacological effect, 59, 69

Psychopharmacology, 21, 51–59

Psychosomatic idea, 15, 16

Psychotherapy, 15

Psychotropic effects. *See also:* Medicaments

Purgatives, 23, 32, 61, 63, 85

Purslane, medical use of, 77

Pythagoras, 30, 133

Regimen of Salerno, 67

Renaissance, medicine during, 16, 19

Rhazes, 25, 99; *On the Repulsion of the Harm of the Nutrients*, 25–26, 97

Rhubarb, medical use of, 20, 85

Rose, medical use of, 131. *See also:* Oxymel of roses

Royal disease, 27, 107

Royal Society of London, 8

Ruby, medical use of, 99

Rufinus, 20

Rufus of Ephesus: *The physician's questions to the patient*, 43

Saffron, medical use of, 125

Samuel, the physician, 115

Sandalwood, medical use of, 65

Saul, *King*, 107

Senna, medical use of, 85, 105

Sephardic Hebrew script, 35

Shlamovitz, Naomi, 53

Silk, shredded, medical use of, 109

Silver, medical use of, 24, 91

Sleep, 24–25, 30, 51, 59, 71, 93, 131, 133, 141, 145; center, 25

Spices, in diet, 30, 123

Spleen, 20

Steinschneider, Moritz, 11, 22, 97, 98, 155, 157, 158, 161, 215

Stomach, and disorders of, 16–17, 21, 32, 61, 71, 73, 85, 89, 113, 135

Sugar, 124, 133

Superfluities and residues, 15, 20, 47, 53, 59, 93, 127, 131

Sweat, 14–15, 30, 83; insensible and sensible perspiration, 83

Syncope, 26, 28

Syria, use of oxtongue in, 57

Tabarzad sugar, medical use of, 28, 99, 111

Talmud, Babylonian and Mishnah, 32, 115, 133

Teicher, Avishai, 73

Temperament, 26, 31, 44, 57–61, 89, 91, 99, 103, 107, 143; hot, 16, 20, 27, 67, 105, 111

Tené, David, 8

Texts of the treatise: Arabic, 165–189; reference to, 7, 9, 12–13, 17, 32, 35, 113, 155–163; English, 41–153; ref. to, 13, 17, 113, 149, 162, 163; German, ref. to, 12, 15, 17, 147; Hebrew, 40–152; ref. to, 7–8, 9, 11, 17, 31, 34–38, 105, 111, 127, 129; Latin, 191–212; ref. to, 9, 17, 25, 35, 57, 93, 101, 111, 150, 198–199

Therapeutic rules: against much fat in the diet, 119, 123; against polypragmasia, 21, 71; against strong purgatives, 23, 85; awareness of possible changes in the patient's condition, 83, 95; awareness of side-effects, 32, 55, 57, 85, 89; compatibility with the patient's constitution or condition, 65, 79, 95, 150; properly organized instructions, 25, 32, 61, 75, 87, 95; testing, 30, 57, 97, 117, 127

Theriac, medical use of, 27, 97

Thrombosis, 99; idea of in Galen, 14

Tibbonides (Medieval translators family), 13

Thyme, medical use of, 23, 87, 105

Toledano, Shula, 8

Transactions of the American Philosophical Society, 13

Translations of the treatise, referred to: Hebrew, 9, 11; Latin, 9–11; German, 12; English, 13

Urine: excretion, 20, 53, 85, 139; clearance, 53

Vajda, Georges, 158–160

Vapors, 15, 32, 51, 75, 83; black, 20, 25, 63, 93; smoky, 14, 20, 53; ascent of, 75, 83, 149

Venesection, 14, 23, 87–89

Vesalius: *Fabrica*, 99–98

Vienna Latin manuscript, 11, 25

Villanova, Arnold de, 99

Vitamin C, 121

Vomiting, 77

Water-balance, 14–15, 31, 147

Water lily, medical use of, 23, 85

Watson, Gilbert: *Theriac and Mithridatium*, 27

Whey, medical use of, 85, 89

Wine, medical use of, 15, 20, 29, 32–33, 51, 53, 55, 57, 59, 119, 125, 152

Zaitchek, David V., 8, 69, 216